MAGGIE COMPORT

Surviving Motherhood

Ashgrove Press, Bath

This edition published by
ASHGROVE PRESS LIMITED
4 Brassmill Centre, Brassmill Lane
Bath BA1 3JN, UK
and distributed in the USA by
Avery Publishing Group Inc.
120 Old Broadway
Garden City Park
New York 11040

Originally published by Transworld Publishers
as *Towards Happy Motherhood*

British Library Cataloguing in Publication Data
Comport, Maggie
Surviving Motherhood. – 2nd ed
1. Women. Postnatal depression
I. Title II. Comport, Maggie
618.7

ISBN 1-85398-013-7

Grateful acknowledgement is made for permission to publish excerpts
from:
An Introduction to Marital problems © 1986 by Jack Dominian:
William Collins Sons & Co Ltd (Fount Paperbacks)
Dealing with Depression © 1984 by Kathy Nairne and Gerrilyn Smith:
The Women's Press Ltd
*Depression After Childbirth: How to recognize and Treat Postnatal
Illness* © 1980 by Katharina Dalton: Oxford University Press
Depression: The Way Out of Your Prison © 1983 by Dorothy Rowe:
Routledge & Kegan Paul Books Ltd
Motherhood and Mental Illness © 1982 by Academic Press Inc
(London) Ltd
Our Bodies, Ourselves © 1971, 1973, 1976 by the Boston Women's
Health Book Collective Inc: Simon & Schuster Inc
The Birth of a Child: the Estate of Dr Grantly Dick-Read

Bound in Great Britain by
Kadocourt Ltd, Aylesbury, Bucks

For Prunella, who has great wisdom, strength and warmth, and without whom there would have been no happy birth. And for Daniel, who is simply wonderful.

ACTION PLAN

If you are feeling distressed and disturbed after the birth of your baby, or suspect that someone you are close to has some form of postnatal depression, turn to the pages listed below to help you understand what is happening and to find out what you can do.

This book contains a wide variety of information and everyone will use the book differently, according to their needs. Some sections offer a way of dealing with postnatal distress; other sections can be read more leisurely with a view to gaining insights into the problems women have postnatally or, hopefully, avoiding them. If you have particular interests, look in the contents, index and appendix to find what you want.

Forewords

Motherhood has always seemed to me something to be proud of and to enjoy – which is also what comes across from this book. But, as it goes on to explain, there are often practical and emotional difficulties to contend with, and the period after birth ends up being very miserable for some women. However, we are never alone in our mixed experiences after birth. My mother's advice on having children was always to remember that, whatever I am going through, I am not the first.

She went through nine births and remembers them as the happiest times. So I was determined to enjoy becoming a mother. Although I was often very tired, had work and money to think about, and various worries, I was too much in love with each of my two babies to allow myself any negative feelings and I think this is a key way of avoiding postnatal depression.

During my pregnancies I talked to both of my babies. Then, when they were born, I cherished each moment, especially the first time I held them, seconds after birth. Nothing was too good for them as far as loving was concerned. I was lucky to have great help from my mother and husband, but then I was never too shy to ask for help or to admit if I had run into difficulties.

I kept my babies as close as possible. At night their place was in my bed or in a cot right next to it. In the day I would either sleep while they slept or put them on my back, African style, leaving both hands free for whatever. Babies feel comforted in this position by the body warmth and familiar heartbeat and don't cry. I liked the closeness of having a baby asleep on my chest in the afternoons. It reminded me to relax, forget all the things waiting to be done, and just treasure my infant.

Patti Boulaye

This book about postnatal depression is of great importance and value because it offers a comprehensive survey of all factors relevant to this commonly occurring and serious condition. The content and format of the book is determined by the fact that it is written for our contemporary society and culture, many members of which are urgently and deeply in need of access to the wisdom and love which pervade this book. The notable amount of work which has gone into its writing ensures a gratifying attention to detail which makes it valuable both as a reference book and as a practical guide to an isolated depressed mother on the point of giving up what she sees as a hopeless struggle.

The book is written, as it should be, by a woman, a mother who has not suffered from postnatal depression, but who sees with total clarity all the factors, obvious to women, which contribute to depression postnatally – factors of which men can and do remain perversely unaware. A perfect example of this blindness in face of the obvious is the male inability to see, to even think, that the current depersonalisation and desexualisation involved in hospital births could have anything to do with postnatal depression.

This book could assist many professionals to escape their professional and institutional rigidities and see things with the penetrating clarity and compulsiveness of the well-born one minute old baby. It could also help all the non-professional helpers of postnatally depressed women to see their roles and responsibilities more clearly. Please read it.

Desmond Bardon, MD, FRCPsych
Adviser to the National Childbirth Trust
Member of the Association for Improvements in
Maternity Services and the Association of
Radical Midwives

Contents

xii

Acknowledgements

For the assistance they have given me in preparing this book, or the inspiration or practical help they have provided, I would like to record my grateful thanks to:

Barbara Baker, Belinda Barnes, Jan Barnett, Beverley Beech, Daphne Bichard, Colin Brewer, Prunella Briance, Agnes Burns, Edith Cansdale, Leon Chaitow, Ros Claxton, Vernon Coleman, Katharina Dalton, Pam and Dave Darby, Clare Delpech, Gaye de Jersey, Jack Dominian, Sandra Elliott, Di Farley, Mary Field, Caroline Flint, Ellen Goudsmit, Pat Gray, James A Hamilton, Sara Heath, Gwynneth Hemmings, Dora Henschel, Yasmina and Edward Henty, Sophy Hoare, David Horrobin, Kathy Hughes, Anne Jenkins, Joan Jerome, Sheila Kitzinger, Pauline Markovits, Leonard Mervyn, Jean Monro, Amelia Nathan Hill, Margaret Oates, Jo O'Farrell, Janet O'Sullivan, Andrea Pound, Kaleghl Quinn, William J Rea, Diana Riley, Ellen Rothera, Sheila Santamaria, Richard Seel, Sheila Simmons, Janet Stephenson, Peggy Thomas, Shirley Toms, Gillian Waldron, Liz Waumsley

Introduction

This book investigates postnatal depression of all forms and puts forward help for mothers. I was drawn to write it because of the contrast between my own good, depression-free birth experience and what happens to many other mothers. After the birth of my son I was filled with energy and happiness and was shocked and saddened to find that PND of some degree was taken for granted by medical staff, pregnant women and new mothers as an almost inevitable hazard of birth. It seemed to me unnatural and unnecessary that such a wonderful happening as birth could result in so much misery and the waste of precious, irreplacable, potentially joyous months with the new baby.

PND is taken for granted yet, paradoxically, no one appears to know for sure what it is or what to do about it by way of prevention, alleviation or cure. Indeed, there is a lack of medical and public interest in the condition, despite it being the commonest complication of childbirth, affecting some 15% of mothers moderately seriously and up to 80% in a lesser way. With over three-quarters of a million births this year in the UK, for example, that is a lot of women involved.

These figures merit more attention and questioning. Either the label is misapplied or something is radically wrong with childbirth in our society – probably both. How can a normal event so often have an unfortunate outcome, one that can have a detrimental effect on the baby, the interaction between the mother and her baby, the mother's relationship with her partner and their whole family, in addition to the mother herself?

It is not known if the number of women affected represents an increase in incidence, absolute or of cases recorded, because comparatively little has been done to study PND. Amazing conflicts of expert opinion exist as to prevalence, degree, form, origins and treatments. Perhaps this is not surprising when professionals concerned with mental health have yet to agree about depression in general.

Many questions remain unanswered; others are still unasked. Some of the things that remain unresolved are:

- What could be causing the prevalence of such a negative state?
- Are more cases being identified rather than more occurring?
- What is meant by 'PND' – used loosely to describe everything from a fit of tears to severe psychosis?
- Is the label being misapplied?
- Could all forms of PND be usefully divided, as in typical depression, into endogenous (without apparent cause) and reactive (a response to something obvious and unpleasant)?
- Does the diagnosis conveniently allow society to evade tackling serious human and economic problems that new mothers suffer?
- What are the effects of the way women now experience birth?
- As hormonal imbalance is implicated, can stress and faulty nutrition be triggering and compounding hormonal problems, preventing the body righting itself?

Is the issue of PND being confronted and, if so, in what ways?
It seems that a greater will to take action is required. For instance:

- Why are so few hard facts available about such a statistically important occurrence?
- Why is the condition accepted with a shrug of the shoulders?
- Why is so little done to help mothers? (Can you imagine post-executive appointment depression being ignored?)
- Why is the help that is offered so useless or patronising or alarming in its implications, social and medical? (Antidepressant drugs and psychiatric help for 10% of women who have recently given birth must be tackling the wrong end of the problem.)
- As further government-funded help is unlikely to be forthcoming, or may be unsuitable if not harmful, can women help themselves in any way?

There is at least a greater recognition that PND is real. Women with the symptoms used to be told to pull themselves together as there was nothing wrong with them. But often nowadays, in a well-intentioned effort to validate women's experiences, so much is done to reassure them that their reactions are not imagination or malingering, that women are coming to believe that it is normal to be depressed postnatally, to have the short-lived blues if no more. Equally, in the important effort to make public and reduce through socioeconomic measures and changes in general attitude the unnecessary stresses of motherhood, so much is being made of the (supposedly) dreary awfulness of being stuck at home with children that mothers may expect to find their babies depressing instead of being open to enjoying these new small people.

Some of the above questions are beyond my resources to answer adequately. Some of them may be as well answered by a mixture of proven facts, personal observations and experience and intuition as by expensive research projects that could be based on false premises and contain inherent biases. What is certain is that new knowledge and understanding cannot be gained without first making speculations that intuitively link existing facts. One of the greatest scientists advised this approach to moving forward. Einstein said, 'There is no logical way to the discovery of these elementary laws. There is only the way of intuition based on Einfühlung [sympathetic understanding, empathy] in experience.'

This book does not dwell on the well-covered aspects of PND. It is about less considered perspectives, origins and answers. It is also the only book on PND so far to deal with all the major possible causes of PND and relate them to each other. In it, it is clear that I support a broader way of looking at PND. Instead of one view excluding others, more progress could be made if we learn to see all views as complementary and partial truths about the whole.

Maggie Comport

In this book:

- When PND appears in the author's text it is used to embrace all types of emotional and mental disturbances and illnesses occurring postnatally. Puerperal psychosis and 'the blues' are self-explanatory; postnatal depression means non-psychotic or 'neurotic' depression which has a wide range of severity. In quoted references these distinctions are not always clear.

- The quotes and references used are not intended to represent or convey the overall and complex viewpoints of any professional or to summarise their life's work.

Chapter 1

What is postnatal depression?

Postnatal depression is nobody's baby. Because of extreme specialisation in the medical profession, mental and emotional disturbances after birth, like the new mother herself, do not seem to be the responsibility of any one group. The training of obstetricians merely touches on PND, they are unlikely to know the mother as a person at all, and their care usually ceases when the mother leaves the hospital. Paediatricians care for babies and children, not the mother, even when her depression is affecting her child. Midwives' responsibilities are chopped up into antenatal clinic, labour ward, postnatal ward, and community work. The GP may not have looked after the mother during her pregnancy, or know her very well, and usually sees her once postnatally at six weeks. Psychiatrists, who will only see a woman after she becomes obviously disturbed, may or may not regard depression in the postnatal period as a separate entity. Either way, it is rarely serious by psychiatric standards, it does not lend itself to easy categorisation of symptoms or causes, and it mostly clears itself up in time.

Postnatal mental and emotional disturbances are very difficult manifestations to pin down, describe, understand, deal with, cure or even improve. Studying them does not bring glamour, kudos or rich rewards. They are a vague woman's problem, and women are notorious for their vague problems, but seem to rub along without anything too much being done about any of them.

Nevertheless, to their great credit, there is a body of doctors who feel scandalised by the hopeless misery of so many women and their profession's neglect of this area. Some 20 years ago American Dr Hugh F Butts wrote, 'The paucity of adequate clinical investigations into the psychiatric ills of women in the period after childbirth is amazing in the light of the gravity of these conditions and the catastrophic effect . . . upon the unfortunate family.'

1

Professor Ian Brockington of Birmingham University's department of psychiatry says of PND, 'We are largely ignorant of its causes and the best way of helping the patients.' And of the puerperal psychosis form of the illness he says, 'In the last 120 years only the hereditary element and the lifetime tendency to mental illness have been amply confirmed.' Dr R Kumar of the Institute of Psychiatry in London says, that 750,000 births a year 'allied to an incidence of about 10% for postnatal depression add up to a substantial problem. Virtually nothing is known of the consequences, if any, of neurotic disturbance in childbearing women.' Professor Brockington and Dr Kumar have contributed to and co-edited *Motherhood and Mental Illness*, 'the first book to review the whole field of mental illness in pregnancy and the puerperium in a comprehensive way.'

To try to counter the lack of information the Marcé Society was founded in 1980 by a group of British and American psychiatrists. Now with a broader membership, it hopes to 'advance the understanding, prevention and treatment of mental illness related to childbearing,' and has already managed to encourage a new awareness of and interest in this problem.

The Society for Reproductive and Infant Psychology was formed in 1983 in the belief that 'The development of the psychology of reproduction and infancy has been retarded hitherto because it has been pursued within the confines of different medical, psychological and other specialities.' Their many areas of concern include 'conception, pregnancy, labour and delivery including preparation therefor, postdelivery recovery, neonatal psychology, early parent-child relations, postpartum psychological disturbance and mental illness, motherhood, fatherhood and marital relations, obstetrics and gynaecology including psychological aspects of surgical procedures . . .' They now provide a successful forum for an interchange of ideas between obstetricians, paediatricians, psychiatrists, midwives and psychologists, as well as other professionals interested in this area.

Most publications for pregnant women, and most childbirth classes, either ignore the existence of PND, or dismiss it in a few reassuring words, often describing only the mildest form and neglecting to mention the possibility of longer duration, later onset or symptoms of terrifying severity. It is left to organisations like the National Childbirth Trust's postnatal committee and the Association for Post-Natal Illness to explain to mothers what can happen and what help may be available.

Getting recognition, understanding and help is difficult, with women either being told that they are not ill at all and should pull themselves together, or that PND is almost inevitable and best treated with drugs. In the NCT's *New Generation* a member sums up the picture. 'The mothers . . . unless they are lucky, are subjected to a quite intolerable burden of scepticism, patronising attitudes, ineffectual treatments and social ostracism, quite apart from their own inherent feelings of guilt, utter inadequacy and total isolation in the throes of an illness which society has chosen to ignore.'

One leading obstetrician and gynaecologist, whose book *Pregnancy* is treated like a bible, epitomises an established professional approach. Dr Gordon Bourne obviously thinks that pregnancy, birth and motherhood are stressful to the point of being overwhelming, not a life event that women can take in their stride. 'Most doctors and midwives consider an attack of "the blues" is almost essential to relieve tension after delivery.' (What on earth did they *do* to the mother?) 'Some emotional disturbance, together with the "postpartum blues", is present in varying degrees in almost every woman who has had a baby.'

So, motherhood equals madness? Such an attitude carries the seeds of a self-fulfilling Catch 22 philosophy – to qualify as a normal woman you must demonstrate you are disturbed. If shows total misunderstanding of healthy changes – the mother's heightened sense of perception, intense happy emotions, excited anticipation and protectiveness of her child. On the other hand, describing disturbance as usual allows real illness to be dismissed as trivial, inevitable, 'just hormones' and self-righting, instead of consideration being given to underlying social and economic factors, previous psychological scarring, plus the effects of interventionist birth.

Dr Desmond Bardon, adviser to the NCT and formerly consultant psychiatrist in charge of a mother and baby unit, views postnatal disturbances quite differently. In the NCT booklet *Mothers Talking About Postnatal Depression* he says, 'It is totally unacceptable for professionals to say, as they are now starting to say, that depression after childbirth is "normal". If by normal is meant "that which commonly happens" then there is something seriously wrong with today's management of childbirth and with attitudes towards childbirth and the sooner the modes of management of and social attitudes towards childbirth are altered the better. If by calling depression normal the professionals are suggesting that it doesn't matter then they are either speaking from ignorance or they are lying. In either case they are wrong.'

The only thing that is clear is that there is a great lack of knowledge and understanding about PND, among medical people and parents. Because of set professional attitudes, plus lack of general interest, we are left with major questions about the nature of PND. There is no agreement on what it is, who gets it, why they get it, how to treat it or how to avoid it. It is not even clear if PND is an illness itself or actually a symptom. Mothers may have no idea what is happening to them, what the experience of PND is like for other mothers, or the beliefs held by professionals who deal with women who become disturbed in the postnatal period.

'THAT'S HOW IT WAS FOR ME . . .'

One reason for the wide professional disagreements on every aspect of PND is that it manifests itself in so many ways. Mothers describe everything from vague unease to not recognising the wild creature they had become, and feelings which are diametrically opposed – 'I couldn't stay awake' . . . 'I couldn't get to sleep'; 'I lost all interest in life' . . . 'I felt wild enthusiasm'; 'The baby was the only person I could relate to' . . . 'I was utterly indifferent to her needs'; 'I felt so lonely' . . . 'I longed for total peace and seclusion'. Following the commonly accepted subdivisions of PND into the blues, postnatal depression and puerperal psychosis (see later) makes patterns of changes a little clearer. Whatever form PND takes, there is no disagreement about the distress it causes.

The blues

It might be supposed that a postnatal ward would be a calm and joyous place. But often the atmosphere is edgy and tearful – 'we were unprepared for the weeping and wailing' said two medical researchers. Mothers say they went through a bewildering range of quick-shifting emotions in the first few days after birth. They shifted from high to low in seconds, felt incredibly vulnerable and over-reacted to everything. They sometimes also were worried by what they did not feel.

4

Louise 'I was amazed at how little feeling I had, how disconnected I was from the baby. Despite already having two small stepchildren, mothering did not come naturally. I didn't feel at all maternal and was terrified what to do with this creature. I cried a lot in that first week.'

Susan 'The third day after my baby was born I felt an overwhelming sense of responsibility, of no longer just being myself but of having another human being I would be tied to profoundly for ever.

'Instead of the father sharing things I could almost see into the future that I would be the one with the "load" to carry. Although I was thrilled to bits at having given birth, overwhelmed with joy to see my daughter and hold and love her, I had at that time an unnerving depression about having become a mother. My life had changed irreversibly, my freedom seemed to have vanished, I had taken on a life-long commitment and it frightened me.

'At the height of my gloom, which manifested itself in floods of tears bordering on hysterical crying, I relived flashes of the difficulties I was having with my marriage. Realisations of my husband's drinking problems, knowing that I would *have* to work to support the family – all these things seemed too much on that day.

'I remember the nursing staff telling me that it was very common to be weepy on the third day. They were very supportive and suggested that I didn't see visitors during my "gloom". This helped and after about 24 hours I began to feel stronger again and able to face everyone and the business of being a mother. I don't think that I'd ever felt so down before and I haven't since.

'It was as though I had no control over my feelings. Suddenly I was rock-bottom, after having been so high at the birth. I hadn't expected to feel this way. It would certainly have helped a lot if someone had warned me that these "blues" could happen.'

Postnatal depression

A shared feature of many mothers' recollections is that they did not realise what was wrong with them and they bitterly regretted the wasted time.

Vickie 'It's all fine and well thinking you're going to have a little baby, but you don't think what's going to happen afterwards. From the beginning, after going home, things went wrong. With a lodger there

5

was a constant merry-go-round of work, pleasing other people, catering to their needs. I was coping 24 hours a day with a wakeful baby plus keeping the house immaculate. I felt rejected by my husband who would go off to the pub.

'After four months it really began to sink in that something was wrong. I felt angry and resentful of my husband and the baby. I began to hear and see things – including a friend of mine who had died. When the baby was about eight months old I tried to suffocate him. I phoned the health visitor and she came round immediately. She said I had postnatal depression and lots of mothers experience this, but no one suggested why or went any deeper.

'The GP gave me antidepressants and these really, really helped. Then I saw a community psychiatric nurse. She listened to and accepted me as I was. Afterwards she put forward some suggestions on how I could change my life. I began to see that an awful lot of surviving is acceptance, but at the same time knowing what you are getting yourself into, saying "This is right for me, I'll do it." At the time she was my lifeline. If I had had only the tablets with no follow-up I would be in a mental home by now.'

Sandra 'I remember smacking my children on their bottoms a lot. I lost two years of their lives that I should have enjoyed.'

Rose 'I look back at that period of my life with amazement and some sadness that so much time was spent in a daze and by a totally different person to my normal, happy, confident and easy-going self. It was like two people standing side by side – me and that awful, weepy, neurotic being which I could not quite get back inside myself and conquer.

'I felt trapped in a web of nervous anxiety, unable to cope with even the simplest shopping expedition. I would feel tense and in a whirl. My mind would go blank. I would just sit or stand, unable to make decisions, as if weighted down by lead. When things got too much I wanted to retreat into a dark, warm, cosy hole. If I forced myself to overstep my limited confidence, I felt physically ill. From my first wakening, my stomach would churn and I would feel in a nervous agitated state.

'Conversations would be left in mid-air, and I would hear voices inside my brain. A complete feeling of madness would overtake me and I would wonder if I seemed all right to other people. How could this possibly happen to me? I went through bleak dark days of depression with seemingly no light at the end of the tunnel.'

6

Lucy 'It probably began actually in hospital. The baby was screaming because there was no milk in my breasts and I stood in the nursery shouting "horrible baby, stop crying" while a student nurse watched in horror. It was a cry for help that went unanswered and I just went downhill for a year.'

Pat 'I used to drop with exhaustion, but didn't realise it was not normal. The doctors more or less said motherhood is exhaustion. I was like a zombie . . . those years were lost.'

Connie 'I hated myself, I felt so guilty. I knew there was no reason. I had a good baby, a good husband. He wanted to help and was very positive, but I just wanted him to accept how I was.'

Alex 'I was afraid to seek medical help, or ask the family. I could not admit I was not coping. The problem wasn't the weight of the responsibility – it was simply too much work. I couldn't have cared less about my husband. He was upset but I would have liked to leave him as well as the baby. I regret missing out on that early time. I couldn't cry when I was depressed. It came out talking to friends in the end and I turned a corner.'

Jill 'Because I was put on a hormonal drip my ability to be in control was taken away. The birth happened too fast and I cried and moaned at the end of the delivery with *real* grief, a real sorrow, total and depressed. There were people around me but I felt terribly alone and abandoned. I hardly registered if the baby was a boy or girl and asked the staff to take it away. Eventually I needed to pee and could feel the hormones draining out of me. There was a sense of relief and everything changed dramatically in my head. I wanted the baby immediately – they couldn't bring her fast enough. I luxuriated in her and felt cocooned with her.

'When I got home I felt peculiar. I started cleaning because I felt the place had to be right for the health visitor. I had lots of little fixations and wasn't functioning in an organised way. When the baby was three weeks old I forgot her outside a shop. On clinic days I would go up to the health visitor a lot. At home one day I tore all the lower kitchen units off the walls. It felt good. When my husband interrupted me I said, "I wanted more light".

'Life was a hurdle all the time; all the time I felt "brace yourself for the next thing". There was no period of tranquillity. It was like everything was in my head. The thoughts never stopped. Everyone was once-removed; I felt once-removed from being a mother. I carefully avoided any relationship with anyone who would tell me about the state I was in. I kept up a good front; nothing was detected.

'By about 15 months I was able to detach myself from the baby enough to stop breastfeeding and by about 18 months I was all right again. I didn't decide until later that I'd had postnatal depression. Now I think it was a process of undergoing necessary changes and was inevitable as there was so much unfinished business going on in my life.'

Puerperal psychosis

Dramatic symptoms means that this rarely goes undiagnosed, and mothers may feel calmer again relatively quickly, but they are usually left with the nagging question – why did it happen?
Linda 'I was one of those rare birds who started flying with the pethidine two hours before my daughter was born and kept on flying until, to the despair of all those around us, we were locked up together for a month in a psychiatric unit. Much postnatal illness goes unrecognised, but when you believe that your baby is the second messiah in female form, you do tend not to be ignored.

'I had experienced manic illness before and therefore was much at risk of puerperal psychosis, although the medical profession did not warn me that was the case. From the champagne, flowers and hilarity of hospital, and discharge home, I was waiting increasingly impatiently for the party of all parties to begin. Every communication, including the radio, was secret messages to me, and sleep became life-threatening. My husband cared for the baby as I entertained the rest of the world, after they had worshipped the miraculous infant. Two weeks after the birth our GP's attempts to inject me with Largactyl to force me to sleep were seen as murderous but experienced as ineffective. After I was hospitalised it took huge doses of Largactyl daily for three weeks to ensure a six-hour sleep.

'Three weeks after we were admitted my baby was attacked by another acutely ill mother who saw her as being possessed by evil, and we all knew that I had to come out. The terrible guilt and pain of having subjected my baby to the possibility of that attack gave me the strength to demand my discharge.

'Women do get better from postnatal illness. Drugs and drugged sleep was the only way that I was going to get better, and it is dangerous to be dismissive of drug treatment in such circumstances.

In a strange way I believe that I was fortunate in having an acute episode rather than a debilitating long drawn out experience of not coping very well. The fear of going mad will doubtless remain with me for the rest of my life.'

Samuel 'When my wife became ill postnatally, to us it was like a knife which suddenly dropped out of the sky and landed sharply between us, separating our closeness. I still don't really understand from where or with what purpose that cold knife came.

'I remember now sensations loosely attached to isolated incidents – all seemingly set in a long, dark tunnel: the abrupt onset of completely unpredictable changes in attitude, the waves that came and went with alarming rapidity; the relentless inevitability of succeeding waves and yet the utter unpredicability of what they might bring with them. This was a sweet, gentle woman who suddenly blew hot and cold, spitting and tearing things apart, raging at those closest to her, trying to destroy materials or people or feelings of love and attachment, feelings of security; and alternating this with episodes of deepest intimacy and tenderness, to be hastily followed, once she was lured into this state, by events such as attempting to walk across the path of an oncoming juggernaut.

'There was the colourless coldness that surrounded her, the visibly altering texture of her facial skin as a wave started to build up again. What hidden force made her attempt to jump from a car window while it was overtaking on the motorway? I remember trying to hold her back when she was jumping from a window 12 metres above the ice and snow; waking in the middle of the night to find her at the bottom of the bed trying to tie the telephone wires around her throat; how she was perpetually terrified into a cowering state by her own thoughts from within; the vacant look in her eyes as the storm would temporarily recede leaving behind an exhausted and bewildered mind; my returning home from work to find the house totally empty and the front of the car stove in. And above all I remember her utter lack of concern about the episodes that was almost as frightening as the violence itself.'

Mary 'We failed mothers are labelled, via the disease known as puerperal psychosis, with madness. Yes, we are mad – mad with anger and rage. My first baby – I loved her enough to cuddle and nurture her, I hated her enough to kill her. These emotions lived together in me.

'The birth was a series of interventions, I was alone, my baby was removed as soon as she was born. This birth left me feeling I had been tortured and raped. It was the most nasty, violent experience of my life. Naturally, one doesn't hold out much love for the rapist – in my case a healthy baby girl. I also had an incredible anger towards my spouse for letting this happen to me. Rape, outwardly a sexual abuse, inwardly has more to do with a violent domination of one individual over another. As a mute mother, totally brainwashed and dominated by medical intervention, I felt I had been forced to surrender my body to their interference. This was done for the supposed benefit of my baby; I was just the passive vessel – they made her dominate me.

'The acceptable thing to say about PND is that the mother couldn't cope. She may even *fear* hurting her child. But I will dare to say the unacceptable thing for my violated self – I would have *loved* to have enacted my anger and killed my baby. The only reason I felt so evil towards the baby and my husband was that I was denied the emotional satisfaction of birth, and birth is a truly emotionally satisfying event if the environment for birth is in harmony with the mother's body. The innate mother in me was all but destroyed by the inappropriate care in labour.'

PROFESSIONAL ARGUMENTS

From the fourth century AD there are references to women becoming disturbed and even mad after childbirth, but the subject was first written about 'scientifically' in France by J E D Esquirol in 1845 and by the psychiatrist Louis Marcé in 1858. The idea of puerperal insanity as a separate mental illness did not receive much further attention for a long time, perhaps because any prevalence of what we generally call postnatal depression was masked by the 'confusion, delusions and hallucinations' which indicated the onset of blood poisoning after birth – a frequent occurrence. By the time basic hygiene, then semi-sterile conditions surrounding birth plus effective antibiotics had dramatically reduced cases of septic poisoning, psychiatrists were preoccupied with schizophrenia.

Even if academic interest in a separate entity of postnatal mental illness had waned, its existence was recognised by the state. The Infanticide Act 1938 reduced the penalty for a mother who causes the death of her child while it is still under one year old from that for murder to that for felony if, at the time, 'the balance of her mind was disturbed by reason of the effect of giving birth, or on lactation'. It was also accepted at a practical level in the forms of mania and melancholia. A 1944 midwifery textbook urges the nurse to keep a special watch for the warning signs of puerperal insanity, 'which usually appear in the first two weeks ... Insanity is commonest after eclampsia, with severe puerperal infection, in epileptics and after a pregnancy of fear and worry.'

Studies in the early 1960s showed there was an increased risk of admission to a psychiatric hospital in the first three months after childbirth. In 1968 psychiatrist Dr Brice Pitt published the results of a long-term study of puerperal women. His finding that 'at least 10% of women giving birth are troubled by postnatal depression of at least moderate severity' attracted interest in the psychiatric profession. Research was also going on into the effects on babies and children of early separation, or of maternal indifference, and into the incidence of child abuse. Links began to be made between PND, bonding problems and 'difficult' children.

During the 1970s there was a move back towards the idea that postnatal depression was a disorder specific to the postnatal period and caused, somehow, by the childbirth process. This school has gradually divided into three main streams as to what about childbirth causes mental disturbances – hormonal changes, inability to cope psychologically with motherhood, or the social and economic stresses of caring for small children. But, there is still a group of professionals that maintains depression and psychoses after childbirth are really no different to those mental states brought on by any other crisis or stress.

While there is at least a greater degree of interest in helping mothers with PND there is disagreement as to how best to do so, because there is no consensus on definition or prevalence. Postnatal can mean from day one to two years. Estimates of how many mothers suffer vary from one in 1000 to 80%. The Maternity Alliance say, 'Postnatal depression affects almost one out of every eight women to some degree after the birth of their baby,' but in 1971 the Boston Women's Health Book Collective said in *Our Bodies, Ourselves*, 'What little research has been done suggests that over half of all women who bear children experience a marked degree of emotional upset in the weeks and months following childbirth.'

The differences in incidence can be partly explained in terms of varying criteria in different studies, partly by the inclusion of surveys of retrospectively self-reported PND, and partly by the timing of interviews. When later follow-ups are done, the incidence of PND can be high – 60% at one year (Frommer and O'Shea 1973), 38% at two years (Raphael-Leff 1982).

With regard to the varying criteria applied, 'postnatal depression' is a blanket term, used to cover 'a range of afflictions from sadness to suicide', says Dr Katharina Dalton, a GP and gynaecological endocrinologist and one of the National Childbirth Trust's panel of advisers. In *Depression After Childbirth: How to Recognize and Treat Postnatal Illness* she adds a fourth category – exhaustion – to the usually accepted subdivisions of postnatal depression. 'It is convenient to divide the afflictions into four groups; maternity blues, postnatal exhaustion, postnatal depression and puerperal psychosis. It is important to recognise that these four groups can merge imperceptibly with each other.'

Maternity blues

Figures for the incidence of this vary, but are all high: 'About half of all women after childbirth' (Dalton), 70% (Harris 1980), 'one half to two-thirds' (Pitt), 80% (MIND). With its occurrence so frequent, the blues are referred to as 'normal' and dismissed as of no consequence. 'It is said that every new mother should experience "the blues". This is a period of fairly acute depression which starts for no apparent reason and disappears for no reason. It usually lasts 12 to 24 hours, generally between the third and sixth day after delivery.' (Bourne)

Sydney Brandon, professor of psychiatry at Leicester University, says in the *British Medical Journal* 'Weepiness is the outstanding feature, usually accompanied by despondency, anxious feelings often related to convictions of maternal incompetence, and subjective impairment of memory and concentration . . . No treatment other than reassurance and support is required for the condition is usually mild and always transitory.' He feels that women who get the four-day blues will be 'none the worse for it'.

Over and over again the blues are shrugged aside as nothing. Few efforts are made to establish if they could be avoided, if the tears of misery should have been tears only of pure joy. As well as being an unpleasant and possibly unnecessary experience, marring the first days with the baby, it seems the blues do have a further significance. It is usually accepted that the direct cause is upset hormones (without questioning why it has become 'normal' for them to be upset), but the blues are likely to have a link with later depression, especially puerperal psychosis. GP Dr Ronald Playfair found that a specially severe attack of the blues on day four was one factor making women more at risk of developing depression.

It may be that today's managed birth can be regarded as a physical/biochemical trauma, no different from any other form of 'surgery' in its depressive effects. Midwifery tutor Valerie Levy used a maternity blues questionnaire to check the postoperative reactions of a variety of patients. She concluded that the term maternity blues seems to be a misnomer as the incidence of symptoms of disquiet was almost identical (maternity 57%, gynaecological 57%, female surgical 59%).

Postnatal depression

This middling group of postnatal disturbance includes everything other than the blues or psychosis, so it is not surprising that this is the category over which there are most conflicts of learned opinion. It starts later than the blues – 'in or after the third week of the puerperium' (Brandon), 'any time during the first year after the baby's birth' (Dalton). It goes on longer – sometimes only a few weeks, often up to a year, by which time 60% have recovered. It is usually regarded as self-limiting, though in some cases 'the changed personality and life-style may persist for 20 or more years' (Dalton).

Although an incidence of around 10% is most quoted, Dr Walter A Brown of Yale University says, 'an untold number [of mothers in the postpartum period] suffer from incapacitating but less dramatic disturbances which often go unrecognised.' Various studies have found rates of 3% (Tod 1964), 14% (Kumar and Robson 1978), 16% at week six, 22% during the first year (Watson et al 1984), and a 36% rate for 'ill-adjusted women' (Breen 1971).

All that can be said for sure is that depression, of some degree, is common after birth. Dr Dalton says, 'The majority of women suffering from postnatal depression do not even recognise that they are ill. They believe that they are just leading a lower quality of life bogged down by utter exhaustion and irritability – a sadly changed character.'

Tiredness, clinically described as 'undue fatigue' but recalled by mothers as 'total exhaustion', is definitely the most outstanding feature of postnatal depression and is dealt with further in Chapter 3. The exhaustion may really be a mild form of depression. Or, it may actually be uncomplicated physical exhaustion. However, the latter, if not ended quickly by sufficient rest (usually unobtainable) will cause biochemical changes that result in depression.

The list of symptoms for postnatal depression is wide-ranging – extreme fatigue, lethargy, tearfulness, anxiety (often related to the baby), panic, tension, general disquiet, despondency, indifference to the baby, guilt, feelings of incompetence and inadequacy, inability to concentrate, remember or think clearly, headaches, general pains and feelings of being unwell, insomnia, early waking, loss of appetite, loss of sexual interest.

One common symptom is a very low flash point. Extreme irritability is a marked and notable feature of postnatal depression, often leading to aggressive outbursts and total loss of control. It is not a symptom usually present in typical depression. Many women describe the feelings as like very bad premenstrual tension and Dr Dalton finds the presence of irritability further evidence for a hormonal basis for postnatal depression.

Opinions on how mothers with postnatal depression can best be helped vary enormously, according to what is thought to have caused the illness – what its nature is supposed to be (see later).

Puerperal psychosis

This extreme condition is rare, affecting only one or two in 1000 mothers, and is clearly distinguishable from other forms of PND. Professor Brandon says, 'The final and most dramatic condition is one in which a few nights of insomnia may herald a florid psychosis with hallucinations, delusions and confusion . . . Onset is unusual within the first 48 hours, but in about 40% of cases symptoms begin within a week of delivery.' Elsewhere it was found that 65% of puerperal psychoses started within two weeks and 94% within four weeks of birth (Protheroe 1969).

Psychotic depression is usually marked by morbid anxiety about the baby, followed by profound despair and guilt. To those who are around her, the psychotic mother can turn into a deranged, alarming stranger, sometimes intent on her own destruction or that of her baby. According to Dr Pitt, a high proportion of puerperal psychotics exhibit mania which 'takes the form of unrealistic over-confidence, brittle gaiety and abundant misdirected energy. The baby is at risk of neglect or mistreatment because the mother is busy doing nothing or has idiosyncratic ideas of childcare.'

Arguing against attempts to classify the symptoms of puerperal psychosis under various other headings of mental illness, American former professor of psychiatry Dr J A Hamilton says, in *Motherhood and Mental Illness*, 'Illness in the puerperium presents itself as depression, mania, delirium, or with delusions and aberrant thinking resembling schizophrenia . . . some patients may move from one constellation to another, or display symptoms from more than one constellation at the same time.'

Hospital admission is usually recommended, preferably with the baby to avoid damaging separation. Most authorities feel that mood-altering drugs or electroconvulsive therapy are the only short-term answers, perhaps with psychotherapy once the main crisis has passed. Dr Kumar says, 'There is a general consensus that puerperal psychoses have an excellent prognosis.' Although recovery rates are high, and more favourable than for non-puerperal psychoses, figures vary according to the criteria applied. Unfortunately, recurrences are common, about 20% for each succeeding pregnancy with the likelihood of a higher risk in women with more severe psychoses, according to a summary of six studies, while Dr Pitt says '50% of puerperal psychotics with a normal life span will suffer at least one non-puerperal relapse'.

Conflicting opinions

The arguments about the nature and causes of all forms of postnatal mental disturbances are endless. This is hardly surprising because, as Professor R E Kendell of Edinburgh University says, 'Psychiatrists have never been able to reach agreement about a system of classification of depressive states. It has been the subject of furious controversy fifty years ago and the arguments have continued without pause ever since.' Ellen Goudsmit is a psychophysiologist specialising in psychoneuroendocrinology and a psychotherapist who has a particular interest in PND. She says, 'There is no generally accepted definition of postnatal depression, no diagnostic test and none of the symptoms is specific to this disorder.'

PND is variously considered as:

- a specific entity with a spectrum of severity
- three separate forms of postnatal mental illness
- a form of reactive depression (due to some external situation)
- a form of endogenous depression ('created within')
- a symptom of hormonal disorder
- a symptom of general biochemical problems
- not an illness, but a realistic response to social stresses

It is obviously not possible to cover the complete and complex views of every professional mentioned in this chapter. The comments that follow are brief, mere samples that serve to indicate what a wide range of opinions is held about the nature and causes of PND.

Dr Kumar finds that, although there is clearly a raised incidence of depression postnatally, 'What is not at all clear, however, is when postnatal depression becomes ordinary depression on the time scale after delivery, and whether there are any special clinical or other features which distinguish postnatal depression from episodes of depression at other times unrelated to childbirth.'

Merton Sandler, professor of chemical pathology at Queen Charlotte's Maternity Hospital, London, has worked tirelessly to get PND recognised as a disease in itself. He says there appear to be definite chemical changes in the brain and has been involved in research to provide a better understanding of these.

Dr Hamilton believes it is harmful for PND not to be regarded as a separate entity. 'When the classifiers of psychiatric illness expunged "postpartum psychosis" from the official list of diseases, early in this century, cases of mental illness which arose after childbirth were distributed into other categories. This action seemed rather harmless at the time . . . In retrospect, it would appear that fragmentation of "postpartum psychosis" had led to the overlooking of many characteristics which distinguish postpartum illness from other varieties of illness. Possible disease mechanisms and possible treatment modalities may have been overlooked.'

Dr Hamilton considers that the following sequence is what leads up to PND. The worries, discomfort and pain of pregnancy and birth are usually followed by relief, happiness and a sense of accomplishment. When disconcerting symptoms occur instead, physical illness seems to the mother the first explanation. When doctors 'reassure' her this is not so, she turns to other possible reasons for her symptoms – she fears they may represent 'incompetence', failure as a mother, or 'mental illness'. 'The interpretations provide fertile soil for the growth of the great variety of psychological aberrations which are so characteristic of postpartum psychiatric illness.'

Dr Bardon says, 'It is now generally agreed that there are no specific mental illnesses related solely to pregnancy, childbirth and the puerperium and that the mental illnesses which occur in relation to these events are essentially the same as those occurring otherwise.'

In considering what causes depressive conditions postnatally he says, 'Applying to these cases the formula that breakdown into a functional psychosis results from stress acting on predisposition, one can say that the genetic predisposition in puerperal cases is easily identified while the stresses are not.

'I suggest that the most frequent and the most important stress factor is psychological, and that it arises from unconscious conflicts in the woman about assuming the role and responsibilities of mother.

'Real or phantasised difficulties between a child and her parents will, when the child herself becomes a mother, be transferred into her relationship with her own child, making her anxious and doubtful about her competence as a mother.'

He considers other important stresses are major life events, social conditions, personal vulnerability factors, loss of independence, and believes there is a high correlation between the amount of technological intervention during childbirth and depression, if this is combined with vulnerability factors.

Dr Margaret Oates, as a senior lecturer and consultant psychiatrist at Nottingham University, balances offering a clinical service for PND with research work. She says, 'My views on the causes of postnatal mental illness are largely drawn from other people's works, but also supported by our own longitudinal research project, in that there is no illness in relation to childbirth which is specific or unique. The overwhelming evidence is that the puerperium, and particularly the first three months after the birth of the child, increases the vulnerability of women to mental illness, but is not a direct cause and effect relationship.

'The overwhelming evidence is that, apart from the fact of childbirth, a family history of major mental illness, obstetric complications and in particular the caesarean section, and a personal history of major mental illness, are the major contributory factors to the so called "puerperal psychosis". The serious illnesses that occur shortly after childbirth do indeed look very different from mental illness at other times, but we feel that this difference is explained by its proximity to the physical events of childbirth and the extraordinary abruptness with which the illness manifests itself – that is to say, not that the illnesses are unique, but merely different because of the proximity of childbirth.

'Regarding the much commoner and milder postnatal depression and other so called neurotic illnesses which occur in about 15% of women, there is no real evidence to suggest that such illnesses are indeed any commoner in the first few months after childbirth than at any other time. In other words, the increase in mental illness is at the very serious and relatively rare end of the spectrum.'

Psychologist Dr Sandra Elliott claims that the traditional theories prevalent in the 1970s led to over-emphasis on hormonal factors and neglect of the various ways in which psychosocial stress can contribute to neurotic depression in the months following childbirth. She welcomes attempts in recent publications by women from various professions to redress the balance by describing the potential for stress, threat and loss in the experiences of birth and parenting and the range of responses women have to these experiences.

Dr Elliott also questions the value of tackling postnatal problems by dividing postnatal women into two groups, PND and No PND. 'Firstly, there are a wide variety of types of psychiatric disorder and psychological dysfunction apparent after childbirth and these demand different theories as well as different treatments.

'Secondly, there is no clear distinction between women diagnosed as having a "mild" neurotic depression and those classed as "normal". All women experience tiredness, stress, tension, anxiety and depression to some degree for some of the time in the early postnatal months, though some much less than others. The two-category approach to understanding postnatal problems diverts attention away from the need to understand what potential stresses surround childbirth and parenting and the goal of identifying which women are in the most stressful and least supported circumstances in order to instigate changes aimed at preventing or ameliorating such depression.

'Thirdly, this simple two-category approach leads to misunderstanding of the complexity of postnatal problems and predisposes professionals without a specialist knowledge to restrict their care of women who are depressed in the postnatal months, such as to the provision of a label and ill-founded reassurances. A caricature of this approach is "what you have got is postnatal depression – it's just your hormones love, it will go away". In contrast, awareness of the complexity of the problem should lead to a more comprehensive assessment of the individual and thereby to treatment appropriate for her and her situation.'

Ellen Goudsmit is concerned that social factors can attract attention away from the underlying condition. In *GP* magazine she says, 'Anxiety and exhaustion can overshadow the depressive symptoms and many women report that their experiences have more in common with a bout of flu than with typical depression . . . Some doctors may fail to notice a mood disturbance in a patient, while others may ascribe symptoms to individual stressors – such as difficult babies, isolation or the low status of mothers in the West. Consequently, they concentrate on these factors as the problems to be solved rather than considering postnatal depression. By the time many mothers reach the consulting room, PND may already have fuelled a family crisis and the resulting deterioration in the marital relationship with its concomitant effects on the woman's health may mislead the diagnostician.'

Professor Brockington and his co-workers put forward evidence suggesting that 'puerperal psychoses can be distinguished from others by their psychopathology' and of studies that 'show striking differences between puerperal and non-puerperal mania.' They also say, 'The only symptom which has so far consistently emerged as "specific" of puerperal psychosis is "confusion" . . . It is embarrassing that the nature of this confusion is so unclear.'

As well as conflicting statistics and schools of thought, there are arguments about whether PND is on the increase, whether it is somehow an illness related to modern times and Western civilisation. When women today recall their own feelings in the period after their children were born, and discuss PND with other women, they report a high incidence of disturbance and depression – 65% in response to questions by the Association for Improvements in the Maternity Services, and seem to feel it is increasingly common. But according to Dr Pitt, Dr Kumar and others, various historical and third-world studies show the incidence of PND stays the same and is not exceptionally high.

Possible origins

Biochemical elements

The various ways in which biochemical problems could be involved in PND are considered in detail in Chapter 4.

In the view of psychiatrist Dr Colin Brewer, 'The causes of postpartum depression appear to be biochemical, but very little is known about the condition,' and he says, 'the genetic element is strong – it runs in families.'

GP Dr EDM Tod in one of his studies found 'anaemia due to either folic acid deficiency, ante or postpartum haemorrhage' in 40% of the cases of puerperal depression. 'It may be that those deficient in folic acid are also deficient in vitamin B6 and that the depression seen in the puerperium results from a disturbance of folic acid and/or tryptophane metabolism.'

Dr Hamilton says, 'Confusion, delirium and hallucinations are now generally recognised as symptoms which suggest that brain function is adversely affected by toxic infection, traumatic or hormonal influences,' and suggests that 'the postpartum fall in oestrogen may be a critical component in the chain of events which initiates postpartum psychosis.'

The best-known proponent of hormonal origins for PND is Dr Dalton but she, in turn, quotes Dr Pitt. 'The presence of confusional features and the absence of personality predisposition or special psychological stresses, together suggest that the syndrome is organically determined . . . the relevant changes might be the precipitate fall in the progesterone and oestrogen levels postpartum.'

Dr Dalton feels that at least 60% of all mothers suffer from some form of depression after birth, varying from feelings of extreme tiredness and over-anxiety to severe psychotic illness. She believes that some individuals are unable to tolerate dramatic postnatal hormonal changes, when very high levels of progesterone drop to insignificant amounts within hours of birth, and that this produces the symptoms of PND. She stresses a high recurrence rate (68%) and the importance of preventative treatment with progesterone for future births where the mother has already had PND.

Social stresses

What part do social factors (marital relationship, male/female status, friends and family, class, money, housing, general environment) play in causing or worsening PND? These factors are dealt with more fully in Chapter 3. Do social factors – trying to be a good mother amidst poverty, poor housing, bleak surroundings and with little support – cause PND, or does PND finally make all this misery intolerable?

In 1978 Professor George Brown and Tirril Harris found a high proportion of mothers of young children were depressed, especially if they were of working class orgin. They listed a variety of social and personal vulnerability factors but concluded that 'it is the meaning of events that is usually crucial: pregnancy and birth, like other crises, can bring home to a woman the disappointment and hopelessness of her position.'

Does marital discord cause PND or does PND cause marital break-down? In *An Introduction to Marital Problems* psychiatrist Jack Dominian of the Central Middlesex Hospital Marital Research Unit says, 'When marital difficulties existed prior to the postnatal depression . . . all that will happen is that an already bad situation will become worse.' In other situations, 'if the post puerperal syndrome is not identified, blame will be laid on the poor marital situation which is interpreted as causing the trouble instead of recognising that the marital difficulties are the aftermath of the post puerperal depression.' He sharply differentiates between postnatal depression and puerperal psychoses, of which he says, 'The prognosis is very good and they rarely play a contribution to marital breakdown.'

In her book *Women Confined: Towards a Sociology of Childbirth*, medical sociologist Ann Oakley focused on the social and medical treatment of women as childbearers and reassessed the meaning of 'PND'. Earlier she had written, 'Science, responding to an agenda of basically social concerns, has provided the label "postnatal depression" as a pseudo-scientific tag for the description and ideological transformation of maternal discontent.' Journalist and writer Vivienne Welburn, author of *Postnatal Depression*, has no doubts about the influence of social factors on PND. 'The monotony, drudgery, low status and isolation of motherhood are delivered to us with the baby.'

Psychologist Sue Sharpe, in *Memories of Motherhood*, says, 'At present mothering, and especially full-time mothering at home, often takes place in conditions that amount to severe social deprivation, where women may be cut off from other adults, from outside interests, from adult conversation and other stimulation, and are potentially vulnerable to depression and other psychological disorders.' Inherent in the work of these women authors is a questioning of the assumption that unhappiness in new mothers is the same as being ill; rather, 'depression' is seen as an understandable response to the stresses experienced.

Motherhood

This role is covered in greater detail in Chapter 3. Changes that occur in a woman because she is dealing with becoming a mother may be misinterpreted as illness. Nearly 30 years ago psychoanalyst, Grete Bibring, in co-operation with a multidisciplinary team including obstetricians, paediatricians and mental health workers, studied the psychological processes at work in pregnancy and the early mother-child relationship. 'They concluded that disturbances were characteristic of pregnancy, not individual, and came to view pregnancy and birth as a maturational crisis, an "intrinsically psychosomatic developmental step" in which biological and endocrine changes bring accompanying psychological disequilibrium which, when resolved, results in emotional growth.' (Boston *Our Bodies, Ourselves*)

Social anthropologist and childbirth educator Sheila Kitzinger has her own views on PND, too. In *Pregnancy and Childbirth* she says, 'All the intense feelings you have during the hours and days after giving birth have a biological survival value for the baby. Without them you would be just a caretaker. Sometimes your emotions are mind-moving and if you had not just had a baby would rightly be thought pathological. But during the first week after birth they are perfectly normal and experienced by many more women than ever openly admit to them.' She also says, 'In fact much of what is usually called "postnatal depression" probably results from a mother's inability to relate to her baby and feel comfortable as a mother because other people have taken over responsibility and it feels to her as if the baby belongs not to her, but the hospital.'

Psychoanalyst and research psychologist Joan Raphael-Leff puts puzzling disparities in predisposing factors or events down to lack of recognition that the same things will affect mothers differently and suggests there are two basic types of women with distinguishing approaches to motherhood. 'To the Facilitator, depression is related to obstacles hindering the pursuit of her new identity and existence as *mother*. To the Regulator, depression is related to obstacles preventing the retention of her previous identity as *person*.' To her, the problems of both types of mother are exacerbated by fatigue, isolation and unfamiliarity with babies.

But the ground for PND is prepared earlier. 'Where original mother-child issues of separateness, primary identification and dependency remain unresolved into adulthood, pregnancy and birth of an infant which catapult the woman into becoming a mother herself, reactivate old privations and endanger established coping mechanisms.' She raises an important question on the way research is done – 'can all women be treated as one group just because they all have experienced a life event in common, namely birth of a child?'

A link with children

Many authorities link childbonding problems with PND. For example, Dr Kumar and Dr Robson (1984) found 'depressed mothers were more likely to express negative or mixed feelings about their three-month-old babies.' However, there is disagreement on whether bonding problems cause or worsen PND, or PND causes feelings of detachment and so bonding problems. Some authorities extend the link to child abuse. Dr Dalton sees a link, Dr Bardon says the child batterers he sees suffer from personality disorders not depression.

Dr Oates says, 'There is no relationship whatsoever between major postnatal mental illness and child abuse, or neglect in the short term, or poor outcome in terms of child competence in the long term. There is a quite strong and convincing link between chronic, minor depression, social problems, delinquency and a whole wide range of socioeconomic deprivation and poor outcome in terms of children's social, intellectual and mental health functioning. It is important to emphasise that women who develop severe mental illness in the puerperium become competent and caring mothers.'

Professor Brockington argues that puerperal psychosis should be distinguished from 'depression complicating the birth of a baby in psychologically painful circumstances (eg when there is a failure of mother-baby "bonding").'

RISK FACTORS

Evidence on what elements in a woman's life could be used to predict whether she is more or less likely to suffer from PND is wide ranging and conflicting, even when careful qualifications are applied by researchers to risk factors they give or discount. The following lists are summaries of a large number of findings. Factors thought to increase the risk of PND are, mostly, what one might expect, but those that have, at some point, been found to have no significance are more surprising.

NOT RELEVANT TO PND

These factors are not thought to have any significant association with the incidence:

- previous psychiatric, physical or obstetric disorder
- depression in pregnancy
- obvious psychological or social factors
- race/culture/nationality
- social class
- number of children
- marital status
- role change
- domestic or financial problems
- individual life events (except bereavement)
- chronic illness in family or woman
- maternal childhood disturbances
- endocrine abnormality
- previous miscarriage
- age
- obstetric complications
- place of birth
- lack of bonding with baby

HIGHER CHANCE OF PND

These factors are thought to increase the risk:
- personal or family history of depressive/psychiatric disorder
- personal or family history of puerperal depression
- depression in pregnancy
- high expressed anxiety at end of pregnancy
- high neuroticism score in personality test
- inadequate personality
- more feminine personality
- excessive compliance
- problems with female identity
- masculine identification
- conflict over assuming mothering role
- prior psychiatric problems in husband
- infrequent sexual intercourse
- unloving, unsupportive spouse
- segregated marital role
- marital difficulties in pregnancy
- being single, widowed or divorced
- no close friends/confidantes
- poor social supports
- over-idealised view of motherhood and feminity
- unfamiliarity with babies
- poor housing/recent move
- recent concentration of disturbing life events
- current difficulties in relationships with parents/in-laws
- lack of maternal employment
- three or more children under 14
- dissatisfaction with leisure activities
- major bereavement in early life
- loss of mother before age 11
- poor mothering/limited contact with mother in childhood
- childhood separation from father
- unresolved psychological problems concerning parents
- envy and hostility in early relationship with parents
- history of two or more years subfertility
- previous abortion
- marked ambivalence about pregnancy
- first pregnancy
- young age
- highly technological birth
- delivery by caesarean section
- birth of a premature baby
- maternity blues

25

Chapter 2

Birth itself

The enormous significance and impact of giving birth is invariably ignored by those who identify and treat PND. How and where the birth happens is usually supposed by them to be irrelevant, but there are many ways in which the experience can have damaging mental, emotional and psychic after-effects.

To most mothers the births of their children are the most important events in their lives, either in themselves or as a watershed. Yet there is general professional disregard for the uniqueness of birth. Emphasis is laid instead on predisposing vulnerabilities – psychological, social or sometimes hormonal. Birth itself is dismissed as merely one crisis that triggers mental breakdown, implying with a degree of inevitability that any life event might have been the last straw for certain fragile individuals. In the opinion of other psychiatrists and psychologists, becoming a mother may have special significance in PND as the critical 'stress acting on predisposition'. But the consensus is that birth itself does not.

Of course, someone who is physically and emotionally in peak condition, has endurance and adapts easily, will stand a greater chance of recovering swiftly and with fewer after-effects from a crisis. But why subject any mother and baby to stress if it can be avoided? No one could argue otherwise than that a gentle, harmonious, spontaneous birth must be more easily gone through by mother and baby than a violent, discordant, forced one. Yet, as a society, we take no steps to increase the likelihood of having a birth experience that leaves good memories, not bad ones. It is as if obstetric procedures have become magic rituals, above question and with a frightful momentum of their own.

To deny the impact of birth itself is to ignore the experience and opinions of mothers. And this general medical denial that the type of birth has any real importance in any way exposes some double-think. For, if the way birth happens is not important, why is it not left to individuals to decide how and where they should give birth? Why the obsession with managing it? Why is birth surrounded by elaborate procedures?

For as far back as we can go in the development of society, and looking at existing societies at a different stage of organisation from those in the industrialised world, birth is definitely not a simple pragmatic matter of allowing a child to be expelled from a woman's body and checking that they are both in good health. Nor is it only a private celebration of loving joy because a particular family has a new member. Instead, the unstoppable life process has been universally ritualised. By whom, and why?

Many births are uncomplicated for mother and child and could progress unaided. But even in unmedicalised societies that rarely happens. It is turned into a social event, and afterwards the woman is regarded by everyone as a different person. Birth is a rite of passage, marking a change in the woman's, and perhaps her husband's, status.

But the rite as experienced in hospitals today seems to have more in common with fanatical ceremonies exorcising devils than with the happy welcoming of innocent, peaceful, tiny new humans. Or the rite in many ways resembles accounts of those dreadful ceremonies where initiates are called on to submit to disorientation, humiliation and physical cruelties, designed to terrorise them into total mental subjugation so that the master of ceremonies may end their old life and, in awesome power and wisdom, create them anew in a mould of his making.

Today's practice does not echo other, more life-enhancing rites. The pattern in these is that, after a period of elaborate preparation and training, initiates are encouraged, aided and supported while completing for themselves some extremely demanding undertaking, calling for physical fitness, muscular and nervous co-ordination, will-power, faith and hope. The completion of this undertaking results in personal growth. It brings wisdom, understanding, deep spiritual insights and an enormous sense of achievement. Completion also results in praise and respect from society. As the ritually changed 'new person' – the mother – then has to care for a totally dependent little person and requires every ounce of physical strength, wisdom, insight, heightened sensitivity and spirituality she can gain, the second model of ritual would seem more appropriate for birth as a rite of passage.

But birth has largely been taken away from those whose bodies house the babies without whose presence the rite would not occur at all. Although the baby's well-being is totally interconnected with the mother's, and traditionally they have been seen as inseparable, modern science enables premature infants to survive in isolation. The baby's welfare is seen as paramount and viewed as separate from the mother's. Parallel with that separation of interests is the view that birth is a messy nuisance and potentially harmful to the baby. Instead of the infant's welfare being mediated through its host mother, short cuts have been evolved to get to the baby direct, the faster the better. Controlled birth is the norm. Vaginal birth is on the decrease. (Well, as obstetrician Robert Sokol has said, 'The vagina is not made for having babies any more than the penis is.')

Women used to know what they dreaded about birth. They could define and describe it and were regarded as absolutely normal and sane to have these fears. Ever-repeated pregnancies, babies getting stuck part-way out, uncontrollable bleeding, infections, were all clear hazards for mothers, not to mention the hazards facing their babies. Now all that is under control. Death in childbirth is extremely rare. But women today do not usually anticipate death at this time. They worry about pain, but cannot discuss it adequately – questions are swept away with 'don't worry dear, we'll give you something.'

Something. What? What do 'they' *do* to you in birth? Every mother says something different, or is strangely unwilling to recall anything that happened. Books are sinister in their degree of reassurance. Commonsense makes any woman wonder how an experience that some friends swear they will never repeat can possibly be something they, in turn, can consider calmly, or remain in control of, let alone 'let happen' to them.

These nebulous but often haunting and overwhelming fears lay the foundations for problems in birth that will necessitate the dreaded interventions, and for emotional and mental illhealth after the birth. To avoid fear, and to remain in charge of birth, means learning more about the natural processes and obstetric procedures, de-mystifying the rites, and questioning how birth happens as it does.

Rites of passage

That modern obstetric practices have a ritual as well as instrumental function is self-evident and well accepted. Richard Seel, ex-editor of the National Childbirth Trust's *New Generation* magazine, looks closely at these ritual aspects in *Health Visitor* and asks 'whether the nature of such rituals may have a connection with postnatal depression.' He believes that in Western society the rites of passage are incomplete. 'This may have psychological and social consequences which contribute to postnatal depression.' He says, 'Rituals can be very helpful to us all – especially in situations of uncertainty or change of social role.' He goes on, 'The rite of passage has three main parts and is only completed when all have been performed.'

Separation This involves removal to a special place, cleansing, new clothing. Its purpose is, through the unfamiliar, to create unease, a fear of doing something wrong and so a willingness to be submissive and dependent. 'Many parents remark on their feelings of confusion and alienation on admission to hospital.'

Liminal period This is a middle transitional stage 'when those undergoing the rite have no status at all' – how true of birth in hospital. 'During the liminal period they may be subjected to humiliation and strict discipline . . . pain may be inflicted on those being initiated, and the liminal period may be climaxed by some bodily mutilation . . . Again the parallels are clear.' These ceremonies may be followed by a period of waiting. The days in hospital after the birth fulfill this role.

Incorporation 'The final part moves the subject back into the world, but now in her new status.' Seel is quite right that this stage of emergence and recognition is ignored. 'The new mother and father are left in limbo, having to fend for themselves as best they can.'

Purpose of the rites One authority suggests 'that the intense anxiety provoked by the rituals and ordeals can help the individual involved to adapt more quickly and completely to his or her new social identity.' Seel says, 'Western birth ritual separates a woman from her normal environment and subjects her to humiliation and disorientation in a strange setting where she is powerless and in pain. As a result of this she is more susceptible to the teaching she receives during the liminal period . . . After this time she should be welcomed back into society, honoured as a mother, and nurtured and supported in her new status. In this way the obstetric procedures necessary to bring

30

about successful childbirth and the ritual procedures necessary to bring about a successful transition to parenthood should run in parallel. In theory, this mix of science and ritual should produce physically healthy babies and socially skilled parents. In practice it doesn't seem to work so well.' It certainly does not.

Postnatal depression In examining the possible influence of the birth experience, Seel suggests three aspects of how such experiences might contribute to depression. (For how they affect the father, see Chapters 3 and 6.)

Symbolism 'The ethos of the birth ritual, expressed as it is in terms of the symbolism of technology and control, may be profoundly upsetting to some parents . . . For them the symbolism of birth may not be life-affirming, but rather perceived as sterile and mechanistic.'

Message 'Instruction and teaching play an important part in many rites of passage.' But advice on motherhood is usually minimal and frequently conflicting. It is also given and received 'in the context of an emotional and ritually charged episode in the mother's life. This means that what in other circumstances might be dealt with rationally and calmly may become a trigger for anger, frustration or depression here.'

Incompleteness The form of the rite is constant everywhere. It 'has its own logic and its own pattern. If that pattern is disrupted or left incomplete serious distress could result. In order for any heightened suggestibility to have positive consequences, there must be a nurturing and welcoming climax to the rite of passage. Otherwise the participant is left high and dry, with feelings of alienation and distress.'

Are we still primitive?

While arguing against 'natural' birth because it is primitive, dangerous and disgusting, obstetricians continue to elaborate the rituals of hospital birth as if these actions would in some primitive way give them power finally to know the mysteries of birth and control them.

Confusions abound in this thinking. Firstly, natural does not equate with primitive. The way animals live their lives, and the elaborate rituals evolved by early peoples have no similarity. Secondly, what women want from birth, for the sake of their babies as well as themselves, is a gentle happy event. There are many ways of achieving this and the connotations of the words natural and primitive may cut right across the concept of a gentle birth. Thirdly, we are clearly not a primitive society, so why do we act as if we were, turning birth into a complicated, often cruel ritual, designed to take responsibility for the process and the outcome – the child – away from the mother?

To return to Seel's observations on birth as a rite of passage. He is clearly right that there are many parallels between hospitalised birth and primitive ritual. And he is right that the third part of the ritual is missing, with damaging consequences, and implications for the incidence of PND. Having deliberately thrown a woman into a state of fear, then left her in limbo, she is not rescued, supported and respected.

But why do we permit the rites in the first place? Is it not time to question whether the birth rites we have now have been distorted, or should take another form, or whether they should continue at all now we do not live in a primitive society? And isn't part three only necessary because of what has, quite unnecessarily, been inflicted in parts one and two? What twisted minds dream up this vortex of events, sweeping the mother away from the security of her moorings and sucking her down, down? And why is there total lack of understanding that fear has no place at birth?

Rites may well have their value, even now, but they do not have to take bizarre and cruel forms. They can be helpful, and give order and shape to an unknown process, but only when there is informed choice as to what is involved. Not when bland reassurance and the constant blackmail chant of 'You wouldn't want to take risks with your baby' conceal mental and physical violence that is sometimes so extreme it can only be interpreted as fierce hatred of birth and women. (Overheard at the maternity department admission desk of a large general hospital. Young doctor, flopping into a chair after coming off-duty, 'That's my carnage for today.')

There is something terrifying and sick about our birth rituals as described by Seel. When animals give birth, they seek absolute quiet and safety. If disturbed, labour may stop, or the offspring may be eaten or abandoned. Yet we deliberately put women in a situation that creates maximum disruption and anxiety and expect birth to proceed unhindered. Such a repugnant practice of disorientation is surely used to trigger a psychological reaction that will end with the woman being utterly compliant, willing to hand herself over like a package to be undone.

32

The birth process alone, without any social or medical accretions, can fulfil the criteria of separation, transition, and emergence of a changed being. However supportive and close her attendants, giving birth is a journey a woman makes on her own. Even if she has given birth before, each labour is an unknown quantity and involves intense excitement and surrender.

The excitement comes from anticipation not fear, and from the awesome and unpredictable strength of the contractions. The surrender is to what must be allowed to happen, not to a group of people who are trying to do it all for you; to one's inner bodily processes, not to outside intervention. By taking herself through the birth, and welcoming and succouring her infant, the woman emerges as a different person with new insights and huge strength. The process is completed when the woman recognises and accepts who she now is. All this she can do for herself.

The function of social ritual is to enable this passage to be completed without hindrance. Reassuring surroundings, warm baths, massage, fortifying food and drink, dim lights, music, and the presence of chosen trusted loving people are all appropriate rituals that support the woman while minimising intrusive influences. An experienced woman in attendance can encourage the mother to let the birth happen. After the birth and a quiet time together, some formal public presentation of the baby, and welcoming of the new family, would complete the social incorporation.

Another problem with suggesting that there is merit in a primitive-style rite of passage is the implication that the mother is not adult before the birth. True, she will be different afterwards and have grown (or could have done if the circumstances had been favourable), but she may well be a mature person before the birth in which case she will resist attempts to manipulate and take her over. She will find the pressure to hand over authority for her person, her birth and her baby particularly oppressive and disturbing. Her anger is likely to be intense. The present 'rites' might be considered helpful to psychologically infantile females, yet these women more often find motherhood overwhelming and are candidates for PND.

Seel assumes one parallel is not true. When talking of the separation stage he says, 'Pain is, of course, commonplace in labour – though not inflicted by those in charge of the women.' Note, he accurately describes the medical attendants as they see themselves and as women too often come to accept, in charge of the mothers. But

33

pain is unnecessarily inflicted by medical personnel who frequently instigate a 'cascade of interventions' (see later). The general atmosphere of fear causes tension that causes pain, as can internal examinations, induced and accelerated labours, being immobile, lying on the back, epidurals, episiotomies, forceps, stitching and caesarean sections.

So why do all these procedures go beyond the pursuit of safety (arguable or not), beyond tidying up birth (desirable or not), and appear to many mothers as gratuitous, punitive and sadistic? Do women require these rituals or do they leave mothers disturbed, damaged and depressed? Why can we not leave birth alone and play a watching brief?

Primitive societies have rites because they fear the unknown, are trying to master nature. Nature cannot be mastered, only understood and co-operated with. And, while there is still much to be studied, we have gained enormous insight into the workings of the world and of our bodies. As medical practitioners know so much about the birth process, why are they so afraid of it that they must wrap it in elaborate ritual?

Is it because birth is a sensual and sexual act that arouses intense disturbing emotions? Is the gap in approach because obstetricians tend to be men and women give birth? Is it because, once started, the reproductive process has its own momentum and a grand inevitability? And this offends the urgent need to control every aspect of the universe, to dissect, pin down and do to death every last elusive mystery?

Or has it more to do with a need to dissect, pin down and do to death every last vestige of the feared female spirit? However wonderful or desirable it may be to share pregnancy, birth and parenthood, men are vital for fertilisation but not for any other aspect of having children. Is it this knowledge that prompts males to take over birth? Is it anger and fear of rejection, of being unnecessary, of female automony?

Patriarchal thinkers, whether representing the medical establishment or fathers, in defending male authority over birth point to the model of natural and primitive male/female relationships where the role of the male as dominant provider is quite clear. This reveals another anomaly in their thinking. As obstetricians keep telling us when denigrating and abhorring 'natural' childbirth, we are no longer natural or primitive. And, studying wildlife reveals no universal rules about male dominance. Among those species where the male does offer companionship and support to his mate, the females welcome this. But they do not need obstetricians' rites to ensure this continues – it just happens that way.

None of the explanations or justifications stand up. We are back to the question of why we, as a society, indulge in rituals that leave terrible scars upon women and are frequently described by them as 'rape from start to finish'.

Obstetricians who continue blindly with their practices, refusing to consider the effects of what they do and to explore any possible deeper significance of their actions, or their obsession with power and control, can hardly blame those women who start seeing modern medicalised hospital birth as an oppressive rite, designed to condition women to accept a role of subjugation and carry out mothering on paternalistic or capitalistic terms and for the purposes chosen by those systems. Or those who view the present state of affairs as a part of a move, starting in the 17th and 18th centuries with the decline of midwives and introduction of male birth attendants, aimed at taking birth away from women. And they can hardly be surprised if the enormous amount of emotional misery if not outright mental illness that has resulted from doing birth 'their way' is laid at their doors.

Safety and technology

A birth that had unavoidable medical problems throughout may still leave a mother happy and satisfied, yet what doctors and midwives may think was 'a good delivery', the mother herself may recall as 'a bad birth'. This trauma can have effects that continue to mar her new life as a mother, and her whole family relationship.

A gentle birth is obviously easiest to accomplish free from complications but the atmosphere and the way the mother is treated are critical to her perception of the experience. We are not talking here of skilful technology versus death in a bloodbath but of when interventions are used, how they are used, and who decides that they are used. It is a difference in attitude.

One extreme is to regard every birth as a potential emergency and the mother as a sick compliant patient. This attitude implies the greatest of faith in drugs, equipment and procedures that are known to have faults and problems. The other extreme is to regard the labouring woman, unless already proven otherwise, as a healthy adult going through a normal bodily function that is highly likely to proceed well.

The first school justify their procedures with 'safety first' and point with glowing pride to a decrease in maternal and infant mortality. But figures for disease and premature death rates this century follow the same rapid decline as those for maternal and perinatal mortality. The dramatic improvement in both predates many medical advances. It is far more likely that public health measures ensuring proper sewage disposal, pure water and strict control of the manufacture and sale of food, improved housing and urban environments, and adequate intake of varied foods, resulted in fewer early deaths both generally and in childbirth. Access to contraception and the effect of that on the number and spacing of pregnancies has made an enormous difference to women's general and gynaecological health.

Increased hospitalisation is usually put forward as the reason for the decline in maternal and perinatal deaths, but although the two trends have run in parallel there is no evidence that the second is a result of the first. And, regardless of hospitalisation rates, babies born to poor families run twice the risk of stillbirth or early death of those born to the professional classes.

The work of Marjorie Tew, research statistician at the Nottingham University Medical School, published after many years of resistance to providing her with key data, makes it clear that home birth provides a safe alternative to hospital birth for many women and babies. Even when so-called high risk mothers booking for hospital births are accounted for, figures for mortality rates are higher when figures for interventions increase.

Twice as many babies die in hospital to very low risk mothers (eight per 1000 birth) as at home or in a GP unit (3.9 per 1000 births). But there were nearly four times as many deaths linked with hospital births in low risk women, 10 times as many in women at moderate risk and three times as many in women of high risk.

Mrs Tew suggests that obstetric practice in the GP units or at home is in fact reducing the risk associated with childbirth but the interventionist strategies employed by hospital consultants have the opposite effect. She says, 'Unless some other factor can be found to explain these results, they must be interpreted as meaning that most infants do not benefit from active obstetric management and most of those already at high risk benefit least.'

36

With regard to interventions, an American study that compared two matched groups, each of 1046 women, found that intervention rates and problems for hospital as against home births were from three to 21 times higher for various items. This was despite the fact that women who developed complications at home and were transferred to hospital during labour were still included in the home birth statistics.

In the Netherlands, home births are the norm and well provided for, but mothers can choose to go to hospital. Recent evidence showed that 'the incidence of complications arising both during pregnancy and labour was significantly higher among the low-risk women who had chosen full hospital care than among those who had elected to give birth at home – and this was true regardless of [number of previous births].'

Satisfaction in childbirth

It appears that there is no proof that safety for mother or child are grounds for the widespread and indiscriminate use of modern obstetric procedures or policies attempting to hospitalise all births. Indeed, the mothers who have resisted these trends in order to preserve the physical, mental and emotional health of themselves and their babies, and who have been castigated and vilified as ignorant and selfish, are now having their concern proved justifiable.

If hospitalisation and obstetric intervention are not routinely necessary, are they what most mothers want? How satisfied are mothers with this type of birth and what it does to them emotionally? Research into what mothers want was recently done at Hitchingbrooke Hospital under obstetrician Mr Hare. The conclusions were that 'a substantial number of women are positively interested in the concept of natural childbirth, and would use such facilities if they were available.'

A 1983 *Parents* magazine survey, which received nearly 7500 replies, found that 'The overwhelming majority of respondents were in favour of the idea that women should be able to have their babies where and how they choose.' But that, 'Sadly, less than two out of three mothers had the kind of labour and delivery they wanted, despite the fact that 75% of deliveries were normal and 95% had healthy babies.' The replies recorded high intervention rates, little

37

freedom of choice on most procedures, and many complaints about lack of information and the unwillingness of staff to discuss procedures.

Dr Marsden Wagner is regional officer for maternal and child health at the World Health Organisation European office in Copenhagen. He is concerned not only about what is safe in childbirth, but about existing paternalistic attitudes towards pregnant women. 'We are willing to tell a woman that her pregnancy is risky, but unwilling to tell her how risky drugs are . . . to withhold information is to insult the intelligence of women. It is their bodies and their babies and their childbirth, not ours.'

The growing membership of childbirth organisations is evidence that women are not satisfied about their options in birth. Discussion at forums and meetings, plus items in newsletters and journals, record the enormous distress caused to women by what happened during their births, its ongoing effects on emotional, sexual and family life, and what they see as a link with PND.

THE CASCADE OF INTERVENTIONS

One major problem of a better safe than sorry, interventionist attitude, or of any procedure used routinely, is that one intervention, however minor, almost inevitably leads to another. The only way out seems to be to question everything.

All procedures increase anxiety. This can directly affect hormonal output and so interfere with the sequences of changes leading up to birth, increase pain and interfere with the birth. Dr Wagner says, 'As doctors, we have forgotten the most basic principle of medical care: first do no harm. Instead we have adopted the philosophy – don't stand there, do something. This approach is particularly dangerous in pregnancy and birth.'

He quotes a professor of obstetrics. 'Spontaneous labour in a healthy woman is an event marked by a number of processes which are so complex and so perfectly attuned to each other that any interference will only detract from their optimal character – the doctor always on the look-out for pathology, and eager to interfere, will much too often change the physiological aspects of human reproduction into pathology.' Wagner adds 'When this happens such complications may be, and often are, interpreted as justification for the original intervention rather than as the undesired result of it.'

Because birth is such a complicated event it would be impossible in this space to detail all the interconnected effects of unfavourable attitudes and actual interventions, so they have been dealt with in the likely chronological order of their being encountered.

Antenatal care

The ball may be set rolling slowly downhill back in early pregnancy. Antenatal procedures and staff attitudes can leave a mother feeling tense, nervous, angry, humiliated, undermined, worried and depressed. Clinics rarely have continuity of staff and getting clear-cut answers and reassurance on key points is almost impossible. The justification for submitting to all this is again safety. Medical antenatal care is supposed to improve mortality figures. But there is quite a school of thought that believes decent living and working conditions, general health care and, above all, enough money to eat well in pregnancy would have more effect.

Hospital antenatal visits wear down the mother's enthusiasm and confidence in herself, and her resistance to unknown, unexplained, complicated and unwelcome procedures that will happen during labour and birth. She ends up feeling, 'Well, maybe they are right' and 'What can I do, anyway.' One consultant obstetrician and gynaecologist has described hospital based antenatal care as 'the greatest con trick ever perpetrated' and admitted that it alters the outcome of pregnancy in very few cases. Detecting a problem and putting it right are, of course, two different things. Concentrating antenatal care on early-detected high risk cases seems a reasonable compromise.

Unnecessary practices

There are several practices associated with admission to hospital and early labour that mothers would prefer to avoid but which hardly seem to constitute medical interventions. But anything unfamiliar or discomforting may disturb or alarm the mother and interfere with her labour. Separating the woman unwillingly from her birth partner at any stage is cruel. Subjecting her to having pubic hair shaved or even trimmed, suppositories or enemas, wearing uncomfortable gowns that get in the way or will not stay done up, using drapes, caps and masks, strapping her arms or legs down serve no purpose and if retained can only be interpreted as empty rituals. Making routine preparations for connection to an intravenous unit, or actually connecting the mother up 'in case there is an emergency' is alarmist. So is refusing to allow a mother in labour food and drink 'in case we have to give a general anaesthetic'. The resulting weakness and discomfort can combine to lower the mother's spirits drastically or slow down labour. Transferring a woman in advanced labour to a special delivery room increases pain, disturbs her concentration, is un-nerving and disrupts contractions.

Internal examinations

These may be clumsy and ill-timed. Most appear unnecessary. Michel Odent, the surgeon who is in charge of the famous birthing centre at Pithiviers, France, says 'Each time you do a vaginal exam, it is another way to inhibit labour. Each time you make a woman change her chosen position, you stop the labour from progressing.' If an internal is done after the waters have broken, it may introduce infection. Repeated internals have replaced traditional reliance on observable emotional and external physical manifestations of the stages and progress of labour.

Amniotomy

Artificially breaking the waters has been linked in one study to a lack of maternal affection immediately after delivery. It is certainly unpleasant and may cause the sudden onset of strong, frequent contractions that are hard to bear. If it is done too early in labour it will not speed things up. On the grounds that infection may occur if too long elapses before the baby is born, hormonal induction may then be used or a caesarean resorted to. Infection is likely to have been introduced by the amniotomy itself or subsequent internals. Speaking of the early natural breaking of the waters Odent says, 'When the membranes have ruptured, in nine out of 10 cases, labour will start in 48 hours. Wait, be patient. We have waited five or six days. It is important not to do a vaginal exam.'

40

Induced birth

What delay constitutes being overdue and whether the hospital knows when the baby 'should' be born are debatable points. Pregnancies are not identical in length and the estimated delivery date is just that. Hospitals do not ask the length of a woman's menstrual cycle, or listen to her version of when the baby was conceived. (Mother, 'But I can tell you the exact date when I conceived.' Midwife, 'No, no, we don't listen to hearsay.')

Ultrasound scan estimates of gestational age are taken as the bible, although they do not always tally with self-reported, known conception dates. Also, according to one doctor, 'Ultrasound measurements of biparietal measurement seem to vary from hospital to hospital, and machine to machine. Anything from 60mm to 65mm may be classified as 24-week gestation.'

So, a mother may be induced when her baby and her body are not ready. This is done by administering hormones (see accelerated labour). In England in 1982 30% of all babies were born after induced or accelerated labour.

Frequent contractions of the uterus in response to oxytocin stimulation can interfere with uterine blood flow and produce foetal distress. Over 10 years ago W A Liston and A J Campbell found that 'Contractions occurring more often than every two minutes are clearly more likely to cause foetal distress, to depress a baby's Agpar score, and to make it more liable for special nursery admission. Such contractions are more likely to be caused by high-dose oxytocin.'

Accelerated labour

'For the baby's sake' long labours are 'not allowed' nowadays. Long labours may be exhausting and unproductive and finally result in the need for intervention. Or it may be the way a particular woman's body gradually and without stress opens the birth outlet and eases the baby out. There is no clear evidence that routinely shortening labour improves the outcome for mother or baby. Certainly the administration of hormones in the form of prostaglandin pessaries in the vagina or an oxytocin drip affects the natural hormonal levels and balance during labour and may have residual effects.

Even more so than with amniotomy, the sudden speeding up and

41

strengthening of contractions may be impossible for a mother to adapt to. ('The contractions were intense, powerful, relentless – something like having your fingers slammed in the car door.') The harshness and lack of time between contractions prevent a woman breathing through them and recovering between and artificial pain relief usually becomes necessary. Pain is increased because the upper segment of the womb is squeezing down on an 'unripe' cervix – one that has not softened and opened enough. Insertion of pessaries interrupts the labour rhythm and being attached to an intravenous drip means the woman cannot walk about or easily move her position.

Professor Kieran O'Driscoll of Dublin does believe in the active management of labour, but is adamant that no treatment should be given until a firm diagnosis of labour has been made because 'treatment, of any kind, commits a woman to delivery, whether or not she is in labour . . . If the initial diagnosis is wrong, all subsequent management is likely to be wrong also.' To him, labour does not begin until effacement of the cervix is actually completed – it is so softened and stretched that it cannot be seen except as an opening.

Pain relief

Early interference means mothers need drugs to relieve pain. Wagner says, 'drug use in pregnancy and birth is part of an insidious chain reaction'. Drugs have dangerous and unpleasant side-effects. 'So what is safe?' asks Wagner. 'It is true that any drug can be misused but it is also true that a drug that is not used cannot be abused.'

Tranquillisers (see Chapter 5) May be given to a mother who is tense and anxious, but will make her restless and dopey.

Gas and air Can make the mother drowsy and disorientated, sick and dizzy, and slow down contractions.

Paracervical block Offered in the first stage. Constant monitoring of the baby is necessary, so the mother must keep still. She does not have time to 'get into' the contractions and when sensation returns she is likely to need further pain relief.

Pethidine Makes some mothers feel drugged and less able to help themselves through contractions; very often produces nausea and vomiting. Hospitals routinely give doses four to eight times what may be needed, regardless of body weight, differences in metabolism, or individual need. Professor Peter Huntingford in *Birth Right* explains why some women feel cut off and out of control on pethidine. It is common practice to give 150mg pethidine with 25mg Stemetil – a drug that helps relieve nausea and vomiting and reinforces the pain-relieving effect, but seems to cause unpleasant 'distancing' in some women. O'Driscoll regards pethidine as a poor analgesic, often making the labouring woman 'profoundly depressed, introspective . . . completely disorientated . . . and confused.'

Epidurals This form of pain relief has a particularly dangerous list of side-effects which are rarely brought to the mother's attention. The package insert for epidural anaesthetic medicine reads as follows. 'Neurologic effects following epidural . . . anaesthesia may include spinal block of varying magnitude (including high or total spinal block); [low blood pressure] secondary to spinal block; urinary retention; faecal and urinary incontinence; loss of perineal sensation and sexual function; persistent anaesthesia, [abnormal sensation], weakness, paralysis of the lower extremities and loss of sphincter control all of which may have slow, incomplete or no recovery; headache; backache; septic meningitis . . . slowing of labour; increased incidence of forceps delivery; cranial nerve palsies due to traction on nerves from loss of cerebrospinal fluid.'

The injection given in the mother's spine blocks sensation in the lower part of the body so the mother cannot feel her baby being born. She must be attached to a drip for the drug, a blood pressure cuff as a sudden drop in blood pressure is common, and another drip that can be used in case other drugs are urgently needed or oxytocin is required to accelerate contractions that are fading because of the epidural, and a catheter for urination. Toxic reactions may occur if the drug is wrongly administered or given in too high a dose. Relaxation of the pelvic floor can interfere with normal rotation of the baby's head. It is estimated that an epidural that actually relieves pain and has no negative side-effects is managed in less than 50% of applications.

Pudendal block Done for instrumental deliveries, it interferes with the ability to push and makes an 'explosive' birth with tearing more likely so an episiotomy is usually performed. The mother cannot feel the descent and crowning of her baby's head and may feel cheated of this experience.

Most forms of pain relief interfere with the mother's ability to work with the birth process and this can lead to instrumental delivery. The link is particularly strong with epidurals where the forceps rate is

70–80%. All these drugs pass through to the baby, with its relatively small body weight and immature defences. 'Drugged' babies may be sluggish and drowsy, require help in establishing breathing, and have problems sucking and establishing breastfeeding. Dr Conway and Dr Brackbill showed that 'delivery medication causes retarded development in muscular strength and co-ordination, postural adjustment, visual and auditory responses and that these effects continue for at least four weeks after delivery. These findings followed both obstetric analgesia and anaesthesia (pethidine and/or epidural).'

Foetal monitoring

'Foetal distress' is a much heard phrase, though it is not clear at exactly what point changes in heartbeat indicate problems, or what degree of stress a baby is able to go through without harm during birth. What is certain is that the almost universal use of electronic foetal monitoring has been accompanied by a great increase in interventions, especially caesarean sections. If a baby is thought to be in trouble, fast rescue is the obvious outcome. But monitoring is an interference which, in itself and by making the mother immobile, may have a harmful effect on labour. Belt monitors are usually heavy and cumbersome, while the attachment of a monitor to the baby's scalp is likely to cause both mother and baby pain and distress. (One brave obstetrician with a bald head suffered severe headache for four days after attaching a foetal monitor to his scalp to test if it hurt.) An added disadvantage is that staff tend to watch the monitor instead of the mother, and trust the frequently unreliable machines rather than their own judgement.

Freedom of movement

Moving around during labour and staying upright while giving birth shortens labour, decreases pain and reduces interventions. An upright birth position increases the size of the birth outlet by up to one third. Lying on the back in labour compresses important major blood vessels and means the baby has to be pushed 'uphill' to get out. In spite of the many proven advantages of freedom of movement mothers are still told to stay in bed and what position they must adopt for birth. When a mother is drugged she may be too dopey to move, and attachment to monitors or IV drips, or having an epidural, means she cannot move. Acceleration, episiotomy and instrumental delivery increase when a woman lies on her back with her legs up in stirrups. She is also deprived of seeing her child being born and perhaps helping him out with her hands.

Timed second stage

Where the second stage of labour has lasted longer than half an hour without signs of progress, some obstetricians regard this as prolonged, undesirable and grounds for intervention. Many women are exhorted and bullied through the second stage with orders to 'push, push harder'. The uterus is a large, complex and extremely powerful bundle of muscles. If it is rhythmically squeezing the baby out of its own accord, little or no effort from the mother with her other muscles should be required. If the baby is not coming out quickly it is frequently because the lower uterus, cervix, vagina and perineum are not yet ready. Anyone who needs evidence that birth can happen without violence and effort should watch baby after baby, unaided, sliding smoothly out of completely calm mothers in the Brazilian film *Squatting Birth*.

Rushing the second stage results in ignoring and upsetting the spontaneous rhythms of contractions, holding then forcing the breath, battling to push the baby out instead of relaxing to open up and let it out, and perineal damage. Odent says, 'The risk of tear is much less without someone giving orders. If her shoulders are supported, the muscles of her thighs will be relaxed, and the birth will be easy. The best way to prevent problems is to give the mother-to-be the possibility to be spontaneous, not to give her orders. Let her express her emotions freely.'

Instrumental deliveries

Because of earlier interventions the mother may be unable to give birth unaided, resulting in a forceps or vacuum-assisted delivery. The mother may be too tired, miserable, drugged, lacking in sensation, or

45

in an unfavourable position. In the *Parents* survey, 20% of mothers had a forceps delivery. When delivery is aided, episiotomy and anaesthetic will be required. The anaesthetic may be wrongly timed or ineffectual.

Episiotomies

Enlarging the vaginal outlet with scissors is supposed to decrease the risk of the baby being short of oxygen during birth, avoid later uterine prolapse, and avoid tearing. In the past midwives took a pride in seeing the perineum remained intact. Now episiotomy is routine in many hospitals with rates of 70–90%.

The cut can be ill positioned, badly done, and even more unskilfully sewn up. The stitching may be done without adequate anaesthetic and interrupts the first hour when the mother and baby can be totally involved with each other. Routine episiotomy does not reduce the incidence of major tears, and small tears heal better and cause less pain than stitched episiotomies.

Fear, tension and pain, produced by other interventions, are likely to predispose to a rigid perineum – which is likely to be dealt with by cutting. One midwife says, 'In my own experience as a community midwife, delivering mainly mothers I already know, and usually giving continuity of care throughout labour, episiotomies and stitches are rarely needed. The perineum yields as the baby's head is crowned. It seems to dilate rather like the cervix does, when the time is ripe, and there is no tearing or undue stretching.'

Slow healing or a tight scar can cause practical sexual problems and psychosexual problems for months or even years afterwards (see Chapter 3).

Caesarean section

When all else fails, an emergency caesarean will be used to get the baby out. In Britain the rate for elective plus emergency caesareans is about one in nine; in the United States is has tripled in the last decade to some 20%. As abnormalities in labour could hardly have changed that much, the reasons for performing the operation must have changed. Obstetricians say the trend results from an attempt to improve perinatal mortality and morbidity, in particular for babies with breech presentation, foetal distress and low birthweight; fear of litigation; lack of experience amongst junior obstetric staff in performing difficult vaginal deliveries, and staffing shortages. With regard to foetal distress, it is unclear whether this is being better diagnosed by monitoring or mistakenly diagnosed. Francome and Huntingford suggest that 'the case has yet to be made on medical grounds for a caesarean section rate much in excess of 6% of total deliveries.' Odent does not believe breech presentation is necessarily an indication for a caesarean.

Following a ceasarean section, as with other surgery, the anaesthetic plus general trauma may result in post-operative depression. This is often compounded by disappointment and a feeling of failure at not giving birth 'properly'.

One further, little publicised problem is the possibility of the anaesthetic not working, and the mother being fully conscious and aware during the operation but, because of the muscle-relaxing drug also administered, unable to alert her attendants to her agony. Following a High Court case some 75 mothers who had gone through this experience contacted the birth organisation AIMS.

The women suffered various disturbances and psychological problems – nightmares, terror of hospitals, ruined sex lives and being unable to face childbirth again. One woman completely suppressed what had happened, not telling her GP because she was terrified 'they' would commit her and take away her baby. A common feature was that the medical profession paid no attention to what the women said. One couple were told by a doctor that the experience did not happen. In sharing what had happened the women said it was a considerable relief to have confirmation of the events and to realise they were not going mad.

Managed third stage

Fear of postpartum haemorrhage, plus the overall trend of rushing through birth as fast as possible, has led to a universally managed delivery of the placenta. This is not generally realised. In the *Parents* survey 95% of mothers given drugs to speed up the third stage were not consulted about it.

Old midwifery practice was to cut the cord only after it had stopped pulsating, to allow more blood to pass to the child. The placenta was left to arrive in its own time and any manipulation by external pressure on the womb or traction on the cord was decried 'as stimulation during the resting stage interferes with its normal processes . . . The third stage should be one of masterly inactivity on the part of the midwife.' A South African obstetrician, Botha, found that among Bantu women who continued to squat after birth until the placenta came away of its own accord and then severed the cord, a retained placenta was an extreme rarity and postpartum haemorrhage requiring transfusion never occurred.

Current practice is to give a swift jab in the thigh as the baby's head is born. This injection of syntometrine (part hormonal extract Syntocinon and part ergometrine, derived from a fungus) is used to help the uterus contract and stop any bleeding, but is unlikely to affect excessive bleeding caused by tissue damage or failure of the blood to clot. The drug makes the lower womb and cervix close up fast so, to avoid the placenta being trapped, it is usually 'helped' out by pressure, traction, or urging the mother to push. All these interfere with the mother's response to her newborn baby. If the mother is not touched and the baby is put to the breast quite soon, its suckling releases the mother's own oxytocin hormone which stimulates the womb to contract.

Today, a mother who rejects third stage intervention will bring the establishment down on her head and be given dire warnings of the terrible risks she is running. This is especially true if an earlier birth resulted in intrapartum or postpartum haemorrhage, even when that was clearly attributable to medical mismanagement.

Yet the statistics on which this trend is based need questioning. Firstly, fewer and more widely spaced births to each mother, and improved nutrition and general health have contributed much to safer birth. Then studies on a managed third stage have no valid control group. As with other studies into the safety of obstetric practices, there is no group which is free from interference, and comparisons are made between types of intervention. The practice of induction increases the incidence of postpartum haemorrhage.

Nancy Stewart of AIMS says, 'Postpartum troubles seem to follow the injection that is meant to forestall them.' The known effects of syntometrine on the mother include 'nausea and vomiting; headache; ['going blue']; a dangerous rise in blood pressure which has resulted in pulmonary oedema, cerebral haemorrhage, and detached retinas; cardiac arrest; and lowering of the prolactin levels which may interfere with breastfeeding. Ergometrine has also been associated with a threefold increased incidence of retained placenta, and an increase in secondary postpartum haemorrhage.'

Checking the baby

'Nearly all babies are subjected to the routine suctioning of their nose and mouth "to clear the airway", without regard to whether or not such a procedure is necessary . . . To subject a baby who is breathing peacefully to oral and nasal suction "just in case" is a totally unnecessary assault. Babies who have difficulty in breathing (and it is five times more common in hospital than at home) are far more likely to owe their problems to the use of narcotics and anaesthetics in labour (and/or the reasons for their use) than to a blocked airway, and if this is the case, mucus extraction will not improve the situation,' says midwife and antenatal teacher Sally Inch in her book *Birthrights*.

Newborns are often suspended by the ankles upside down to drain any fluid from the air passages and smacked to startle them into crying. 'Dr Leboyer's photograph of a screaming newborn baby with its fists clenched by its face speaks volumes on the subject of the needless suffering imposed upon the newborn.' Such treatment is also likely to strain and damage the spine and hip joints. Placing the newborn on the mother's abdomen face down achieves postural drainage while keeping him peaceful, safe and warm.

Immediate assessment of a baby's condition, and rating it on the Agpar scale, can be done by simple observation while the baby is on his mother's abdomen or in her arms. Measuring, weighing and further checks are often carried out unnecessarily swiftly, before the mother has had a chance to cuddle her baby and feel he is 'real'. The baby may be taken out of her sight or even to another room.

Special care

If the baby needs help to survive, or special attention, he will be taken from his mother to a special care unit of one kind or another. Some emergencies result from birth interventions – inducing a birth prematurely, the administration of hormones, analgesics or anaesthetics.

Nearly one in five of all newborn babies will spend some of their first hours or days in a neonatal unit.

Having a baby that is especially tiny and vulnerable or is unwell is worrying enough; having to leave the baby in a separate place is heart-breaking; but the rules and regulations and difficulties of access may be the final straw. Yet, more flexible systems have shown to improve the babies' welfare and parents' ability to relate to the child, while keeping a tiny baby on its mother's body the whole time may be a more appropriate way of protecting and nurturing it. Anything that distresses the baby will distress the mother as well as making the child more difficult to deal with and affecting their relationship.

Hospital stay

The postnatal stay in hospital is recommended as an opportunity to check the continued welfare of mother and baby, an opportunity for the mother to rest and recuperate, and a chance for her to be taught how to feed and care for the child. But once emergencies relating to or caused by the birth have been sorted out, community midwives are perfectly able to watch over the new mother and baby at home. Few mothers find noisy, stuffy, unfamiliar hospitals with their inexplicable timetables and disgusting, un-nutritious food the ideal place for a rest while some find their hospital stay positively disturbing. And guidance on feeding and care of the baby, which could more appropriately be offered at home, is often doctrinaire and conflicting.

BIRTH AND PND

What effect do all these interventions in the birth process have on mental states postnatally and in what ways are managed births and PND linked? Our body chemistry can be interfered with directly by chemicals and hormones that we are given; certain physical procedures can indirectly affect hormonal output and balance; and emotional turmoil, fear or repressed anger will produce chemical changes. As our emotions and mental states are mediated biochemically, all imbalances will be reflected in emotional and mental reactions.

The way we are delivered of our babies now can cause mental distress and disturbance directly and indirectly. Many of the contributing factors interact with and compound each other, but they fall into the following general categories.

EFFECTS OF
INTERVENTIONS IN BIRTH

- direct chemical effects on mothers of drugs used in childbirth
- disturbances to hormonal processes caused by induced, interrupted or condensed birth sequence
- biochemical reactions to physical manhandling, instrumental trauma, surgery
- emotional effects of heavily medicalised interventionist birth
- disturbing effects of hospital atmosphere, attitudes and treatment by staff, antenatally, in labour and postnatally
- stress caused by separation from birth partner/s
- anger, as a reaction to what was done during birth, that is unidentified, repressed or not listened to
- insufficient, unsuitable, poor-quality food during labour and postnatally
- cumulative emotional and physical shock at whole unpleasant birth experience
- resentment of and difficulties in relating to the baby as a result of unsatisfactory or downright nightmarish birth experience
- sadness at being separated from a low birthweight or distressed baby resulting from too early induction, the use of oxytocin or other drugs
- difficulties in feeding or relating to a drugged, sleepy baby
- inhibited response to a baby that is edgy, restless and crying because of ungentle birth, clumsy handling or early separation
- problems dealing with a baby that is responding adversely to his mother's alienation, indifference or depression
- lack of uninterrupted peace, privacy and comfort for mother and baby to get to know each other
- exhaustion from dealing with a disturbed or distressed baby

51

The voices of experience

It would seem impossible that emotional distress and biochemical disruption do not contribute to the toll of postnatal depression and psychoses. Yet very little research has been done into the role of the place and type of birth in causing PND. But no hospital based study could draw meaningful conclusions because they would all be comparing like with like – mothers in an alien environment being managed through a process that, in the majority of cases, would proceed unaided. The only differences between groups of mothers used for comparison would be the degree or type of intervention. It is almost impossible to have a hospital birth without interference.

I gave birth fairly recently in a hospital famed for its open approach. Only weeks of questioning and explaining on my part, plus an adamant refusal to agree to any intervention as routine, got me the joyful birth I had hoped for. I was the *only* mother in my large postnatal ward who had *no* interventions. Even then, for the sake of peace, I agreed to certain checks I did not want or believe in, although they did not upset me – two or three internal examinations and limited initial periods on an external monitor (because the particular model gave me some freedom of movement). In spite of my wide connections with birth organisations and a circle of friends and neighbours with babies, I have not yet found *one* other mother who had a hospital birth free from interventions.

Feeling that the effects of gentle, intervention-free birth carry through beneficially into a mother's relationship with her child is not the view only of those few women who do manage to get the kind of birth they want. Nor is feeling that their nameless misery and dissatisfaction as new mothers, or months of clinical depression, or sudden psychotic behaviour, were linked to the sort of birth they had 'merely' the individual subjective conclusion of untold numbers of mothers. Those, medically qualified or otherwise, who deal with new mothers have been convinced for a long time of a link and are concerned that this aspect is ignored when PND is treated, or its possible prevention discussed.

The principal of midwifery education at a major London teaching hospital says she is '100% convinced' that the place and type of birth have an effect on postnatal depression. Caroline Flint, another senior midwifery sister says, 'I feel there must be some significance in the feeling of despair and failure that many women have after a caesarean or forceps delivery and that this might well precipitate postnatal depression.'

One woman who has years of experience running an advisory group for pregnant women and new mothers believes that the physical, biochemical and emotional are very tightly linked and that hospitals have many adverse effects upon the mother and her relationship with her new baby. In pregnancy and immediately post-partum nutritional deficiencies have a marked effect and women's metabolism is particularly susceptible to drugs and hormones.

Either going through an interventionist birth or fighting to avoid it causes stress. The result of this is likely to be a long, tiring, perhaps ineffectual labour, more interventions, and emotional distress. Psychosis may result immediately, or depression after a chain of events. The mother may lose her appetite, produce little milk, have cracked nipples, or poor-quality milk that leaves her baby hungry and yelling. She can become exhausted, lethargic and uninterested in sex. A 'bad' birth puts a woman in poor shape to withstand the social stresses of early motherhood (see Chapter 3) and gives her the worst start to an undertaking that is difficult and demanding, if potentially very rewarding.

General practitioner and author Vernon Coleman says, 'Current medical practices around childbirth are unnecessarily interventionist . . . Women are encouraged to expect childbirth to be painful – by doctors who have turned a natural event into a medical event . . . This leads to much unnecessary worry . . . It is very likely that the pressure put on a pregnant woman will affect her state of mind before, during and after childbirth.'

In 1980 a paper was given at the sixth International Congress of Psychosomatic Medicine in Obstetrics and Gynaecology that made connections between birth and depression. It linked birth problems with 'rigidity of the uterine orifice', which was considered to result from psychological causes, and spoke of 'The considerable frequency of birth complictions [being] followed by some forms of depression . . . The difference between spontaneous births and those with surgical intervention is significant . . . The correlation between course of birth and depth of depression is particularly noticeable.'

Mrs Prunella Briance runs the Dick-Read School for Natural Childbirth and is a childbirth educator of some 30 years' standing. She is dedicated to the concept of gentle, spontaneous, painless birth and is quite sure that the place and type of birth affect the whole process of birth and a woman's subsequent mental state. She says, 'There is no question of PND in a properly handled natural birth.' But, 'If a woman is treated cruelly in birth, this could easily cause postnatal depression.' She also feels that the way a woman is dealt with during labour and birth, and her hospital stay afterwards, leave her shocked and drained of energy and that 'tiredness is critical' in triggering PND.

Jean Robinson, past chairman of the Patients Association and a lay member of the General Medical Council, defends mothers against the charge of selfishness. 'I have just spent two hours with yet another mother who is still having terrible nightmares more than a year after her rapid oxytocin-enhanced delivery, who feels she was technologically raped and whose sex life has been ruined . . . Alas it is amateurs like me and other members of AIMS who have to try to pick up the pieces, since psychiatrists don't seem to recognise or admit the existence of iatrogenic mental illness when it's under their noses . . .

'I learned about women's perspectives of childbirth at the Patient's Association . . . Many letters came from women who had given birth before technology took over and doctors started treating the uterus like a car engine that could be revved up. They insisted they had not been depressed after normal (or even complicated) births where there had been no unnecessary interference, but after this one they were suicidal. That was when I started reading the literature and realised that no one was building into the research assessment of psychiatric morbidity of new procedures, although postpartum depression is now the commonest complication of childbirth.'

The late Dr Grantly Dick-Read, author of *Childbirth Without Fear* (originally published as *The Birth of A Child*), believed that an unsatisfactory birth produced ongoing emotional damage, so 'the further understanding of childbirth is not only of obstetric value.' One of the most important results of 'a good birth' is that 'freedom from fear of childbirth is now justified by experience and the memory of happiness remains where so many recall only unhappiness . . . A high percentage of women in homes for the treatment and care of psychopathic conditions are found on analysis to have a basic cause of their disease in the fear and fantasies of childbirth. Healthy women who have had their babies naturally do not suffer in this way. There is no more health-giving experience in a woman's life than a happy natural childbirth.'

But, when birth was unhappy, women 'start motherhood with a

54

sense of half shame and half disappointment . . . Not infrequently the mother-child relationship is impaired and much of the neurosis that breeds family discord is based upon the frustration that assaults the maternal emotional balance . . . Frigidity and all its underlying fears and inhibitions insinuates the wedge of misunderstanding and irritability or, at the very least, throws a strain on marital loyalty.'

Odent emphasises the role of some of the hormones involved in spontaneous labour and birth and believes hormones also play a key role in a woman's start to motherhood. He says that after a normal delivery, 'when the mother is secreting the right hormones', she is in 'such an intensive state she knows instinctively what to do'. To allow the most helpful sequence and balance of hormonal production he says it is important to arrange a first stage where all sensory stimulation is minimised. Adrenaline production, which goes up when someone is frightened or cold, needs to be limited as much as possible. On the other hand, circumstances need to be favourable to the maximum secretion of 'the hormones which are important as well in acute sexual events, the ones produced by the pituitary gland and known as endorphins. These are like natural morphines, like opium and drugs which can protect us against pain and give a feeling of well-being and induce ecstasy.'

A 'good' birth

Does such a thing exist? Can the event be anything better than 'not too awful'? Is it possible to have a birth that is a happy, positive, enlightening, strengthening experience, one that results in close bonding with the baby and lays the ground for good future family relationships? One that is an act of love and creates love? Yes, if the mother learns enough about birth (see Getting Help), prepares herself for it physically and psychically, and there is reciprocal trust and respect between her, her medical attendants and birth partners.

As the mind so strongly affects the workings of the body it is vital for all involved to be convinced that birth is a normal female function, not a medical emergency. Not so one woman's GP and consultant obstetrician who seems typical of many. Sandar Warshal of AIMS came to the view that 'Nothing in their training or in their practice had prepared them to listen to or respect women. They had little understanding of, or belief in, normal pregnancy. They didn't appreciate the vital link between the total well-being of a woman and a healthy pregnancy. Fear, power and careful mechanical monitoring were their guides.'

If a hospital birth is truly felt to be a wise precaution then everyone at the birth should know and have confidence in each other and the birth should happen in a special birthing room with completely unobtrusive emergency facilities.

Interventionist practice as routine is justified with 'better safe than sorry'. Yet 90% of mothers cared for by Dr Grantly Dick-Read, whose philosophy avoided intervention, had *absolutely* straight forward births, while only 2% needed some interference. Dr Dick-Read found breech presentation no problem and very rarely resorted to caesarean section. This achievement has been dismissed as irrelevant, as has the good safety record for planned home births. Critics say his methods would not work in most circumstances, the women he saw were atypical – healthy, well-fed and housed, educated, highly motivated, personally attended throughout pregnancy and birth by a dedicated doctor with years of practice.

This does not constitute an argument for dismissing Dick-Read's work, or the gentle birth ethic. If critics really believe good results are due to these factors, logically, they should be fighting to increase the safety of birth and decrease the need for interventions by ensuring the good environmental and personal health of all women, providing them with adequate information about their bodies, and giving continuity of care.

In any case, remarkable as Dick-Read's results were, even in today's hospitals some 80% of babies are delivered by midwives, who are seen as capable of dealing only with 'normal' birth and constrained to call a doctor if problems or emergencies arise. By their own standards, obstetricians find that the majority of births don't merit their presence, so why isn't the process allowed to be spontaneous? Safety cannot be the real reason. The reason does not actually seem to be medical (see later).

Midwives' role

The historical decline in status of the midwife, the near disappearance of midwives attending home births, and the ongoing battle over the exact status and role of midwives as independent practitioners must be of concern to all mothers. Although educated in large anonymous hospitals, taught how to use technology and drugs and subject to indoctrination on the advisability of managing birth, midwives are nevertheless the guardians of 'normal' birth. Unless problems arise it is they who attend birth, not doctors, as many people erroneously think.

The profession is asking itself many questions about its role and how it deals with mothers, the most outspoken group being the Association of Radical Midwives. Obstetricians do not seem to be engaged in the same heartsearching and painstaking re-assessments, but then they are not an endangered species.

Midwives as women, often as mothers themselves, and as the people who have most contact with mothers, are uniquely placed to affect a woman's perception of her birth and the immediate postnatal period. Even if, in hospitals, their power to affect the course of birth is limited by the rules laid down by the consultants in charge, they still exercise a lot of *de facto* power.

Odent is a unique male medical voice, because he emphasises the emotional importance of the midwife's role, even to the point of excluding a male presence when that is found to be disturbing. 'I stress the importance in our view of a caring and experienced midwife – the midwife, as a female, is felt to be a caring person. The midwife is a substitute for her mother . . . We have the feeling that the woman needs to be in touch with her own mother; this explains why the midwife is important as a female.'

One of the main barriers for midwives who want to be more involved with, sympathetic to, and 'tuned in' to individual mothers is the hospital organisation that makes continuity of care almost impossible. Caroline Flint, author of *Sensitive Midwifery*, says, 'I do think at the moment the work of midwives is very unsatisfying in that most midwives look after women they don't know and that must be very, very hard.' On the subject of PND she feels that midwives do have special opportunities, certainly to recognise it early on. 'It only seems sensible that if a woman is looked after with love and sensitivity throughout her pregnancy, labour and puerperium it must be helpful. If she is given confidence by her midwife, they compliment her or they encourage her or they acknowledge that she is good at things as a mother, then it just has to make a difference and be useful.'

Expression of emotion

The idea that birth must be managed extends to pressure on the mother to exhibit self-control. If she does not hide her emotions and keep quiet she has failed, she is in disgrace.

A mother may be told she is hindering the birth. ' "Don't scream," the gentle nurse warned me, "or you'll take the energy away from the pushing." ' Usually there is a sharp reminder that she is disturbing everyone else, mainly the staff. 'Down the hall I heard another woman scream . . . "Close the door, we can't listen to that," said my doctor.' (*The Mother Knot* by Jane Lazarre) The venting of justifiable anger at unwanted procedures, loud ecstatic moans, shrieks of joy, even tears of happiness, are included in the ban on self expression.

Sheila Kitzinger has again and again said that labour and birth is a psychosexual experience, put forward the undeniable parallels between birth and orgasm, and pointed out how ridiculous any attempt to clinically manage an orgasm would be, and how surely such interference would adversely affect or stop the process.

As with orgasm, there is a definite connection between parting the lips, whether by letting the mouth fall loosely open or by crying out, and the opening of the vagina and pulsing of the womb, and it is a recognised technique for helping women to give birth spontaneously. In contrast, holding back the vocalisation of emotion means clenching the mouth. This resistance and tension is echoed throughout the body, including the whole birth outlet.

Some women gain energy from crying out. As the martial arts teach, sharply expelling air from the lungs – easiest with an accompanying yell – gives intense strength. Other women make noises because they are totally abandoned to the birth. Odent encourages vocalisation. 'A good transition is only possible when a mother is really instinctive, on another planet, only then can she accept what is not acceptable . . . she can scream freely.' It seems to be this abandonment, with its frankly sexual connections, rather than the actual noise, that disturbs so many medical staff.

Holding back the expression of emotion during labour and birth not only interferes with birth physiologically but begins an emotional process than can lead to PND. Any unfinished business, unresolved conflicts, suppressed feelings, are dangerous to mental health. They fester away and, if not brought out, may result in deep depression which apparently has no cause.

THE BIOCHEMICAL LINK

So, to recap, in what main ways could the type of birth be thought to cause or contribute to postnatal mental disturbances of all types? Unsatisfactory or traumatic birth creates:

- hormonal disturbance = PND
- hormonal disturbance = birth problems = emotional disturbance = more hormonal disturbance = PND
- problems dealing with or bonding to the baby = emotional disturbance = hormonal disturbance (compounded by breastfeeding factors) = PND
- possible damage to the baby = emotional disturbance and/or bonding problems = hormonal disturbance = PND

What is experienced as emotional disturbance is thought by some authorities to be caused by biochemical disturbances, by others to cause biochemical changes. Either way, the role of biochemistry has to be considered. In the case of emotions, mental states and birth, the various hormones are always involved in some way (see Chapter 4).

Birth and power

When discussing birth with women, it is clear that, as mothers, birth partners and midwives, they generally experience obstetric technology as depressing, and this has as much to do with atmosphere and attitudes, with being drawn into a system where one thing leads to another, as with specific procedures. Birth now involves loss of control. Not to one's body. To choose to surrender to and go along with the birth process, to abandon oneself to its physical and emotional intensity, is not to lose control.

Women are deprived of, and in some cases refuse to accept, responsibility for their bodies, their births and their babies. Not accepting responsibility may be a genuine case of opting out. But it is usually part of a vicious circle of conditioning and inadequate information. If you do not know that you have a legal right to control your birth, you do not know much about the physical, emotional or pshysic aspects of the process, you do not know that it can happen any other way, and you simply do not realise what you are letting yourself in for, you will not realise what sort of birth you could have or how to achieve that.

At a deeper level, if you have as a gender been conditioned by society to accept that you are less than adult, and never been given or educated to use responsibility, you will lack the basic mechanisms for gaining power over your life. And if, as an economic class, you have been conditioned to accept that those with education and position know better than you do, you will not trust your own judgement. If lack of money has deprived you of an education that both gives you information about your body and teaches you how to get, process and use information for yourself, you will find it difficult to question what is happening or argue against it.

Most damaging, perhaps, if you have accepted Western 'scientific' devaluation of intuition and instinct you simply will not trust yourself at all (see Chapter 7). Yet intuition has been defined as 'a psychic act, whereby one experiences reality from a true and valuable perspective', and we must learn to heed and trust our inner voices.

If we do not, the nettle that has to be grasped, in the issue of birth and in the issue of mental illness, will be left untouched. The real issue is not science versus nature, but when and why and how technology is ever used and who decides. The nettle is *the issue of power*.

Why women accept such loss of control in birth is uniquely puzzling. Because, for power to be exercised over a woman in birth, she has to consent to deliberately going to a special place, run by a small professional group, where she knows she will be subject to physical handling and procedures and her voice counts for little. In other terms, why do women consent to the rite (see earlier)?

A massive apparatus of psychological conditioning, now so universal as to be invisible to many, is in operation. Those who uphold it are undoubtedly as much under the sway of the circular logic as the women 'patients'. They, presumably, believe they are acting in good faith and in the best interests of women and babies. But there is individual plus organised resistance, with various levels of awareness as to what is going on. Organisations that seek to help women retain and regain control over birth are flourishing (see Getting Help), though some have preferred to concentrate on the arguments about technology versus nature, or seem unaware that this is not the only issue.

The one sure way to weaken any woman's resolve to follow her own wishes and instincts in birth is to say that she may be endangering her baby. It requires massive confidence to say that you are sure your way of giving birth is not only better for you physically and emotionally but is actually safer for your baby. To say that you will accept the consequences of going it alone – even if that is the death of your child. In fact this choice should not have to be made. If maternity emergency services were brought up to a high standard instead of being run down, and well-equipped maternity ambulances plus trained paramedics or 'flying squad' doctors were on call, the risk would be minimal.

However, the whole argument of safety has been misused. As an AIMS journal editorial says on 'the place of death at birth', 'The possibility of death has become so remote as to be almost unacceptable . . . We must not fear death so unreasonably that we impair people's lives in unfounded efforts to avoid it.'

The nettle of who has the final say, parents or doctors or government, has to be grasped because of the immediate and ongoing agony and misery caused to women and their families by birth as it happens now. To have an opinion on who should have power one has to consider why it is presently in the hands it is in, and why anyone would want power over the birth process, anyway.

A *Radical Science Journal* editorial on the medicalisation of birth says, 'Power derives not from medical technologies themselves, but from women's social isolation which makes them vulnerable to dependence on medical procedures in the first place.' And, 'We need to clarify the power relations in women's entire lives which lead them either to demand control over childbirth or accept medical manipulation.'

Individuals cannot be considered outside their social group and that group is subject to wider influences. In that way the personal does inescapably become political in the widest sense. In pondering the problems of an individual, very little thinking takes one on to the subjects of gender and money. Life is different for men and women – particularly because of giving birth – and different for rich and poor. Why it is so, and if there is anything to be done to change matters, in the short or long term, is a matter for individual study and conclusions

– based on improved access to information from as wide a variety of sources as possible.

Women's ability to create new human beings, with minimal help from men if that is how circumstances of social organisation dictate it shall be, makes them very powerful, so potentially dangerous. Historically, this power has been curbed in various ways: by limiting who has access to women to impregnate them; by depriving them of independent economic status; and by appropriating the products of their labours – their children. As least earlier societies had the sense to maximise the chances of the child surviving birth and being healthy by leaving birth alone and taking over the child only at some later point.

Now social control over fertility has crept backwards through birth and pregnancy to conception. Legal rules and medical practices govern the intimate acts of individuals and affect their private family lives. In considering who does and who should control each and every aspect of reproduction, the personal is now definitely political.

To limit distressing birth experiences, and the toll of postnatal emotional and mental disturbance that follows, we have to not only learn more about birth but about the way individuals deal with each other in relationships and the way society works. We have to take more responsibility for our lives.

Chapter 3

Social factors and psychic pain

Conventionally, PND has been seen as an individual problem, and in terms of a woman's failure to cope with or adjust to becoming a mother. This view has been taken without asking whether it is reasonable or remotely sensible to cope with or adjust to motherhood as defined in our society, or in the circumstances in which the woman lives her life, many of which are beyond her control. Deep feelings of guilt are a common symptom of PND and, as the Boston Women's Health Book Collective say, 'We often feel guilty because we think our own inadequacies are the cause of our unhappiness. We rarely question whether the roles we have are realisable.'

No one lives or develops in a vacuum. Everything takes place in a social context. Any methodical consideration of the structure and functioning of human society transforms social factors into sociological ones. Whatever labels we use for the way we live and our lives are run, these are politically organised so what might appear to be individual psychological problems always, on examination, have a political dimension.

Should individuals aim to fit themselves and their children into society as it exists, or change society to accommodate their needs and express their ideals? Whatever path they choose, conflict arises. To imitate role models demonstrated to you, to try hard not to be a square peg in a round hole, may involve damaging manipulation of deeper urges and lifelong suppression of individual needs. To seek for a change in society, even if it does not cause direct conflict with the law, will mean regular skirmishes with all embodiments of establishment thinking, a sense of being an outsider – unsupported and unprotected – and possibly loss of family backing and difficulty in finding a soulmate as a sexual and domestic partner.

It has been suggested that the origin of disease lies in the conflict between society and the individual. Conflict with external forces, or conflict within occasioned by these forces, causes stress. Whether an individual chooses to deal with poverty, rotten housing, an exploitive job or soul-cramping social roles by accepting their lot and trying to be happy within an existing framework, by battling to get out, or by seeking to change the whole system that creates these conditions, there is no escape from stress.

We are designed to cope with stress that comes and goes, and a life without stress would be one without physical or mental stimulus. But unremitting stress, stress piled on stress, causes harmful changes which some authorities would view as psychological and others as biochemical, though the two are actually inseparable (see Chapter 4).

The way to avoid these changes, which result in depression and other forms of mental distress, is to reduce the stress. As certain social factors that cause stress are out of our control, and do not in any case lend themselves to swift improvement, tackling and avoiding as many sources of stress as possible is vital to reduce the total load. So is protecting physical health as much as possible (see Chapter 4 and Chapter 7).

Sometimes looking at some aspect of life from another angle can transmute the energy that was being taken up by conflict into a more positive use. Sometimes merely acknowledging that certain elements of your life are a problem can defuse them as sources of stress. But reaching such insights is hard in the isolation that many new mothers suffer. Changed perspectives are usually achieved after discussions within a trusting relationship with other women – whether friends or professionals.

Recognising what difficulties you face is certainly the first step to mental health. Some of these difficulties are so common and glaringly obvious they become invisible. Through the research of many people, such as G W Brown and T Harris, Andrea Pound and Maggie Mills, Ann Oakley, Dana Breen and Sue Sharpe, the deleterious effects of a variety of social factors on the mental and emotional health of mothers of young children is now recognised. Sadly, academic identification of stressful circumstances has not led to any concerted public effort to reduce them.

It is true that social changes are expensive and difficult to engineer, and may accurately be construed as interference. But a pessimistic acceptance of the status quo is enshrined in current plans to screen mothers, picking out 'vulnerable' (weak?) individuals so that they can be propped up (better conditioned to accept their lot?).

These schemes do offer much needed 'first aid' assistance, but they show that PND is still seen by those who provide funding as an individual problem.

Simply becoming a new mother involves stress because it is something completely different. But this type and degree of stress should be a stimulus to personal development (see Chapter 7). However, if a woman is already struggling to keep her head above water – whether in dealing with psychological problems going back to childhood, sorting out the mixed messages from society telling her what a woman should be, keeping the balance in a difficult relationship, making ends meet financially, or trying to stay cheerful in bleak surroundings – having a baby can be one stress too many.

The situation is exacerbated by the way women are usually required to give birth now (see Chapter 2) and the way motherhood and the domestic role generally are viewed. And the stresses of becoming a mother – intrinsic and socially determined – occur at a time of biochemical vulnerability and readjustment (see Chapter 4), so may overwhelm a woman.

The range of psychosocial stresses which could contribute to a mother becoming depressed postnatally is explored here. Some women take the stresses they encounter in their stride; others will receive adequate support from their partner, family or friends to see them through. But considering what stressful elements could be present in your own life, and not drawing back from examining those that make you feel sad or uncomfortable, or have implications for a change in your life, is worthwhile. Acknowledging deep pain, then permitting yourself to feel angry, are two vital steps in avoiding or overcoming depression.

BECOMING A MOTHER

Whatever the genuine difficulties of domesticity and being a mother, they are greatly magnified by the gap between romantic dreams and stark reality. Images of babies are predominantly beautiful and healthy, either gurgling merrily or deep in untroubled slumber, while the home is warm, luxurious or at least comfortable, and miraculously self-cleaning. That these pictures cannot be more than partially and occasionally true is evident from the most limited and casual contact with any live mother, yet the rosy ambience glows on. The perpetuation of these myths is blamed on the media, the revival of Victorian views about the family, or the continuation of capitalism.

But people have always dreamed, and always found fairy tales about how their lives could be more bearable than obvious reality. Our present insecure circumstances in a declining post-industrial society and under the shadow of the Bomb probably make clinging to charming myths and a romantic view a desirable escape for more women. But there is no evidence that having a safe and comfortable background, or an advanced education that includes studying sad and very realistic literature, stops women choosing to imagine their own lives could be transformed by meeting Prince Charming and be ever after filled with light, love and laughter.

While there is no excuse for the continued presentation of a patently false reality, and especially cynically aiming to make money out of concealing the truth about domestic life and motherhood, you cannot force women to accept a reality they find discomforting and unbearably depressing. In the film *Never on Sundays* the Greek woman played by Melina Mercouri regularly attends the performance of classical Greek plays on her Sundays off. She watches, completely enraptured. When her academic American friend tells her the true meaning of the cataclysmically tragic tales, she becomes enraged. No, no, she insists, he has got it all wrong. They are joyful stories, everyone lives happily ever after.

The Stepford Wives Syndrome

The conscious or unacknowledged manipulation of women's dreams so that they will channel their energy into servicing men and society and not resent their lot is another matter. Whether the role of traditional wife and mother is just the way society has developed, or whether the creation and perpetuation of that role is part of a plot to prevent women claiming what is theirs depends on your point of view. There certainly exists a whole 'Stepford Wives' syndrome.

In Ira Levin's story about the families that move to the lovely suburban town of Stepford, all the wives gradually change. They give up interests that take them away from domestic duties and childcare, keep house perfectly, stop mixing with other wives, become submissive to their husbands and take a great interest in their appearance – becoming mysteriously bigger breasted and more beautiful. In fact the town is a paradise of total male supremacy. The men actually get rid of their real wives, replacing them with humanoid robots modelled on the original women. A chilling fantasy, but expressing a male dream for women who give them no trouble, who are permanently preserved in aspic to service them sexually and domestically and rear their young, and who the men do not have to bother to acknowledge as real human beings with feelings and needs of their own.

Many aspects of male dealings with women covertly or overtly contain a mixture of hate and fear, the desire for a passive, compliant, ego-soothing robot. In so many ways women are seen as objects, not people. What are the implications for women as individuals, partners and mothers in the message printed bold and clear outside a Florida nursing home – 'Bring your wife here for a Caesarean section and keep her passages honeymoon fresh'? This is not an isolated phenomena – 90% of upper and middle class Brazilian mothers submit to Caesarean births largely in the interests of male sexual satisfaction.

Disappointments

While some women, like the Stepford wives, are mainly unaware of the forces at work on their lives, others know in their hearts they are agreeing to a less than fulfilling life yet 'choose' to accept the dreams that are presented. They do this either because they do not feel strong enough individually or as a group to resist the pressures, or they feel at this stage of the game seeking what they want from life will leave them with the worst of both worlds, or because they do not want to accept full responsibility for themselves.

Other women may feel they have an open and equal relationship with a sharing and understanding partner. They may clearsightedly imagine the more difficult and unrewarding sides of being a mother. But none of this is the same as actually being at home with a small baby and living out parenthood. Indeed, the change in lifestyle and loss of control can be as much of a shock for these women as the amount of hard, boring labour can be to a woman who looked forward to playing the traditional maternal role.

For both types of woman the contrast of reality is made greater by the natural absorption of the pregnant woman in herself and her growing baby. During pregnancy women fail to notice or deliberately ignore problems of marital relationships, living conditions or work. They concentrate on the momentous event of birth and are genuinely blind to difficulties that will start or be worse after the baby arrives, or cocoon themselves in the warm satisfaction of the life within, and follow Scarlett O'Hara's well-tried way of coping with grim reality – 'I'll think of it all tomorrow.' But after the birth they do not have the time, energy or money to change their circumstances.

Giving up work

Relatively few people have jobs that are rewarding in terms of interest, sense of achievement, status and money, and women on the whole have worse jobs than men. So pregnant women often view with relief the prospect of time out, seeing a busy new life in front of them, and reasoning that they will not need as much money when they are at home. They will have lots of time to do the things they want to do, and they will keep up with all their old friends.

Initially, at least, not having to go to work is a pleasant change for most mothers. But giving up work – for the duration of paid maternity leave, for the first couple of years, until the children are at school, or for longer – involves a lot of losses as well as certain gains. The losses vary with the nature of the woman's work but include:

- regular contact with adults who share some common ground
- job satisfaction
- job status
- money, both loss to household and loss of personal income
- feedback and praise
- male company and flattery
- casual social contact with strangers through work or travel
- the discipline of getting dressed to go out
- justification for spending money on personal appearance

The loss of independent means is hard to bear, especially when coupled with a family's straitened financial circumstances. Clothes that were worn for work are often totally unsuitable for wearing round the house while caring for a new baby, and the mother may feel particularly in need of a new image, new underwear and a good haircut after the end of her pregnancy, but most mothers are filled with paralysing guilt when it comes to spending money on themselves and not the baby. 'Who will see me, anyway?' they reason. And that can quickly lead to 'I feel such a mess I hope no one sees me,' sealing the social isolation of quitting work.

New responsibilities

Another shock for the mother is the substitution of a job at which she is experienced and competent and for which she may have received elaborate and protracted training for work that she has never done before, may only have read about, and where there are no 'workmates' constantly to hand to show her what to do. A woman who has had one or more children already will know more, but every child is different and coping requires a new set of responses, plus an increased ability to juggle simultaneous crises. Professional teaching, or the advice of other mothers, is conflicting. Much worse, women are not brought up to have confidence in their own judgement and capabilities, and the 'feminine' quality of intuition is despised and distrusted.

The awesome responsibility of caring for a new life may totally overwhelm some women. Although little enough realistic advice on the practical aspects of looking after a baby is available, the concept of preparing oneself emotionally, morally or spiritually to welcome a separate human being is absolutely ignored. A few close families, or strongly religious communities, or access to printed American material on spiritual parenting will sustain some mothers, but most are given no insight into the qualities they will require.

The sheer strangeness of fulltime domestic and babycare routine makes the work hard for a lot of women to come to terms with. Some elements of some jobs will help, but the repetitiveness yet unpredictability, the need to be always alert and infinitely responsive yet to wait rather than initiate, the physical fiddliness of many actions, coping with several things at once – none of which can wait – and, above all, the constant fragmentation of time, energy and tasks are unique to babycare. Neither is it made plain to the pregnant woman that caring for a small baby is a fulltime job – feeding, cleaning, changing, dressing and generally organising a baby can take six hours a day. Housework has to be done on top of that.

Some women plan to throw themselves enthusiastically into the role of creative homemaker after the birth. They imagine the whole place transformed when they do all the things they never had time to do before. But caring for a newborn is not compatible with DIY home improvements or anything else that requires sustained concentration and cannot be stopped, repeatedly, at any point. Some babies sleep very little, perhaps only six to nine hours out of 24, while breastfeeding can take 30 minutes every two hours.

Nor does a programme of intellectual renewal or taking up fresh interests fit in with caring for a baby. Apart from the fragmentation of time, most mothers find they cannot settle to absorbing new information after the birth. This is for the very good reason that new mothers go through a period of change and development and they already have a fulltime intellectual and emotional challenge in their child. Unless a woman realises this, stops feeling she is 'out of things' and welcomes total absorption in her baby, she may find herself both irritated and depressed.

The positive value of early isolation with a newborn and exclusion of other distractions is misunderstood and neglected. There is pressure to rush routine tasks, getting them out of the way as fast as possible in order to get on with 'real living'. This is unrealistic in ignoring just how much time these tasks take up anyway, and the fact that babies cannot be rushed. This thinking does not recognise that absorption in the baby, the constant handling, contact and repetition of routine tasks, provides a way of mother and baby getting to know each other (see Chapter 7).

Love or indifference

Women expect and are expected to feel instant deep love for their babies, and many mothers do respond like this. But for a variety of reasons a mother may feel nothing at all, or be very ambivalent. A traumatic birth, separation from the baby, disappointment about its sex or appearance, marital tension, sheer tiredness, or the stirring up of suppressed emotional pain may all interfere with the mother's response to her child. Depressed mothers have been found to be more likely to express negative or mixed feelings about their three-month-old babies, but it is not known if this is the result of their being depressed, or whether their feelings about their babies caused them to become depressed.

Not being able to exhibit obvious love for a baby is difficult enough to deal with, but the disapproval aroused by this has to be dealt with, too, forcing a woman into guilty concealment of her feelings. This censure is part of society's pressure on a woman to meet general ideals of being a 'good' mother. These are not very clearly laid out, so there are numerous ways in which it is possible to 'fail' to live up to the image.

Breast may be best, but in some circles women can be made to feel a failure and a poor mother if they do not breastfeed. Again, the matter is seen as individual and not in its social context. The pressure is especially upsetting to a mother who has ambivalent feelings about her baby or cannot respond to it. Difficulties with breastfeeding may have physical or emotional causes. An added problem for some women is dealing with their partner's mixed-up ideas about what breasts are for or who should be touching or seeing them. Some men cannot make the switch from viewing their partner's body as private sexual property to it being occupied by, then available to, the baby.

Lack of realistic preparation for motherhood, both the practical aspects and understanding of the way a baby thinks and develops, make it easy for the most loving mother to make genuine mistakes in caring for her baby. If she realises them quickly she can feel wretched that she has caused her baby unnecessary discomfort or actual suffering. If she does not realise them, she can feel the unhappy or protesting baby is unmanageable, presenting insurmountable difficulties, or is rejecting her.

As the situation gets out of hand, the mother may lose control and start hitting her helpless baby, invariably then being overwhelmed with remorse, but often unable to stop a repeat. Many authorities dispute that depressed mothers are more likely to abuse their children, but it does seem likely that acting violently is both an expression of disturbance and something that causes the mother greater distress (see Chapter 6).

Superwoman

The low status of housework and childcare, the assumed boredom of being engaged in domestic and maternal tasks, social isolation and the pressure to be superwoman, doing ever more, ever better, are all linked. If work is considered of value then workers take a pride in what they do and are encouraged to understand all aspects of their job and do it properly. Women's domestic work has never been any harder or heavier than the other kinds of work they were called on to do. Nowadays it is usually looked down on not because it is hard and menial so much as being considered boring.

The daily tasks of housework and childcare are actually no more boring than most jobs. Building a relationship with a brand new human being you have just created is certainly more interesting than sitting on a production line. What is different, and leads to resentment and depression, is that domestic and childcare tasks are performed in isolation, without recognition or thanks, without admiration and without financial reward. And there is no going-home time, no sick leave and no holidays. (One study found that, other than being in paid work, 86% of mothers with a child under five did not have even one hour a week when they were completely free from the responsibility of all their children.) In other words it is the terms of the contract rather than the job that causes the trouble.

Because women are assigned a lower value than men their work is considered to be nothing – any idiot could stay home and keep the family going. If domesticity is so simple and boring, it must be possible and desirable to pack a lot more into life – run a beautiful home efficiently, bring up exceptional children, plus do a paid job, participate in local organisations, go to evening classes, be a dazzling hostess and, of course be an intellectually stimulating, well-informed, beautifully turned out, sexy mistress.

Given the terms of their contracts and the dissatisfaction they feel with home life and babies, many women accept the idea that their work is boring and low value and therefore should not take up much of their time and energy. They either push themselves into doing too much, or feel utterly inadequate because running a home and caring for children takes up all their time. Fortunately, the dreaded superwoman is being systematically debunked, but not before innumerable women have made themselves ill emulating her, or sunk into depression because their lives seem so limited and they feel useless by comparison.

Social isolation

Mothers are not simply pressurised into trying to be superwoman. They often see it as a way of enriching their lives, a way out of extreme isolation. This isolation starts with a sense of anticlimax soon after the birth. There is rarely any formal celebration of the baby's birth, welcome of the addition to the community, or recognition of the mother's changed status. The mother has gone through her long pregnancy with a sense of anticipation. She has, all too often, endured a traumatic birth. Where the baby's arrival is informally recognised, it is the baby that gets visited, praised and given presents. Even that is over quickly and sometimes no one takes any further notice of the mother's pride and joy. The baby becomes another anonymous bundle to be tut-tutted about if it makes a noise in company. Contrary to what the mother has expected, her baby often receives only the most perfunctory interest from the doctor, health visitor, grandparents, other relatives, friends, even its father. The mother and baby tend to be excluded from adult society generally – either by being made to feel openly unwelcome or by the lack of practical provision.

Smaller families and improved standards of accommodation have brought more domestic privacy. When this peace and privacy is enjoyed by choice that is a wonderful improvement on having no space to oneself. However, the very architecture that guarantees privacy reinforces inertia in overcoming social isolation. Other comforts like washing machines in the home, freezers to reduce shopping trips, televisions and videos increase the inertia. Going out with small baby is a performance; why bother when you do not have to?

Women often do not realise how few social contacts they have until they leave work. Families have fewer members and are frequently split up and spread out. Those who travel to work may scarcely know their neighbours and be too far from work colleagues to see them. In any case, the social lives of families do not easily fit in with those who have no children. Travelling to work, or the time taken up by work plus housework, means that working women may not get involved with local activities and organisations. If they have been, continuing previous interests can be impossible with a baby to care for.

Existing friends – couples or single women and men who do not have children – may fall by the wayside, while in some neighbourhoods breaking into the circuit of mothers with small children requires a dedicated campaign. When mobility is limited it may be difficult to discover like-minded souls within a small enough area. Some social classes, ethnic groups or countries have a weaker tradition of female friendship than others. And this social isolation occurs at a stage when women do not necessarily have the time, energy or transport to get out and actively seek new friends and acquaintances.

It is a very depressing experience to have no exchange of conversation all day long, day after day. And new mothers desperately need sympathetic, non-judgemental, kindly friends with whom they can discuss everyday childcare queries and problems, their feelings on the birth, the baby, their partner, their new life as a mother, and the emotional turmoil they may be experiencing. Without ventilation, understanding and feedback these sometimes profoundly disturbing feelings – which should signal a period of growth and development – can be turned inwards to cause mental, emotional and psychological problems (see Chapters 6 and 7).

Returning early to work may provide some mothers with the answer to loneliness. But, assuming she can return to a job she likes, the new mother can feel unexpectedly cut off from her colleagues by the experience of birth, her changed priorities, and sheer lack of free time. Or she may feel guilty and 'unnatural' that she does not want to be with her baby all the time. Finding adequate, affordable childcare is a nightmare for many mothers. Knowing your child is leading a limited life in less than ideal circumstances, but having to harden your heart because that is the best you can arrange, is deeply upsetting and debilitating. Many women return to work early solely because their financial situation leaves them no choice. And some of those are quietly breaking their hearts at the long daily separation from their little babies. There is nothing new about mothers with babies having to work, but spending long hours out of sight and sound of their children, often miles away, is an unwelcome change.

Exhaustion

One universal symptom of PND is described by doctors as 'undue fatigue' while mothers call it total exhaustion. It is no longer medically fashionable for a woman to have a lying-in period after the birth, resting in bed for one to three weeks with the minimum of visitors. Nowadays, a mother will often be moving around within hours of the birth, and may be home within two days or less. She will probably feel well enough to resume some household duties and to entertain visitors.

Much of this energy comes from a biochemical 'high' after birth, and if the mother feels well and energetic it is tempting for her to be very active. But this high evaporates as the body adjusts, and as shortage of rest and broken sleep begin to take their toll on the unaccustomed mother. After an uncomplicated birth very few mothers today are nursed through their first weeks by a relative, let alone a midwife. It is certainly true that being upright and moving around avoids circulatory problems and encourages the body to return to its pre-pregnant state. But totally ignoring traditional wisdom undermines a woman's ability to cope and lays the foundations for deep tiredness that can turn into clinical depression.

'Long uninterrupted sleep is essential during the puerperium, but it is particularly important in the first few days . . . Insomnia is often due to excitement, notably caused by visitors who come too often and stay too long, . . . No visitors should be allowed after 6pm and the best time of all is in the morning . . . After delivery a woman is in a state of emotional instability. She is easily depressed and easily exalted . . . therefore, as far as possible she should be isolated . . . Each afternoon the room should be darkened and quietened in order to allow sleep.' This is the wisdom of a typical 1940s midwifery textbook.

Another benefit of some period of retreat is that it allows the mother and baby uninterrupted time to get to know each other intimately and may result in a more tranquil baby (see Chapter 7). Of course, the freedom to retreat, even partially and periodically, depends on the availability of support for the mother, and nowadays frequently no one is free to provide this except the woman's partner, and he may be ill-suited to the role for practical or emotional reasons. However, unless mothers limit what they undertake and snatch rest when they can, they may find themselves turning into zombies, then becoming disturbed, in a short time.

Though the mother may not realise it because she makes a good recovery, the birth itself can be very draining. The majority of women today have a 'normal' birth, but that description depends on what is currently considered usual. Most births have so many physical interventions that they constitute a surgical operation, after which rest would be advised. In addition, the birth may be emotionally traumatic, but this and the resulting exhaustion go unrecognised. Then mothers are simply not prepared for how tiring childcare is. They expect or are expected to do too much, too soon. Where there are existing children the mother is expected to take the new baby in her stride.

Serious misconceptions exist about the amount of time that babies spend asleep, and at what stage they sleep through the night. Over a third of all parents suffer years of problems with wakeful children. It is bad enough actually coping with a baby that likes being awake most of the time and never sleeps more than three hours at a go without the mother guiltily worrying what she is doing wrong, or searching endlessly for 'the answer', or being made to feel by her partner that it is her responsibility to see he is not woken up. Mothers with two or more children who are awake at different times are in a desperate situation.

Keeping prisoners awake is a classic method of torture, known to lead to breakdown, yet because total exhaustion is so general, it is accepted as inevitable and its prevalence and effects are badly underestimated. The Thomas Coram Research Unit, in studying the transition to parenthood, looked at mothers' health. They found that the scores for minor ailments rose during pregnancy, but by the early postnatal period had regained old levels. 'The one symptom that showed a long-term effect was "tiredness".'

Many mothers who are labelled mentally ill are actually physically drained to the point that they cannot think straight. The effects of lack of rest are worsened by poor eating – with no appetite, no time, no peace and no energy, it is hard to prepare, eat and digest sufficiently nourishing meals to help protect against stress. The problem of shortage of sleep is compounded by broken sleep, and by the earlier sleep problems of late pregnancy. Wakefulness leading up to the birth deprives the mother of rapid eye movement sleep. REM is a sign of dreaming, which occurs in deepest sleep and this deep sleep is needed for physical and psychological restoration. After the birth, when a mother has insufficient sleep and her sleep cycles are constantly, arbitrarily interrupted, she builds up or worsens a backlog of REM sleep loss, which can lead to physical and emotional disturbance.

BEING A WIFE

Having a child does not automatically bring a couple closer together. On the contrary, fresh problems arise and any marital or social problems that existed before the birth are invariably made worse by the introduction of another, totally dependent, person onto the scene. And these problems have been linked with PND, both as cause and effect.

Christopher Clulow of the Institute of Marital Studies at the Tavistock Centre, London, says in his book *To Have and To Hold*, 'In the excited anticipation of life with a baby, it is common for parents to overlook the passing of hitherto important aspects of life as a couple. Yet marriage is changed by parenthood. Changes involve loss as well as gain.' In the book's foreword Dr John Bowlby, honorary consultant psychiatrist at London's Tavistock Clinic, says, 'When a couple have their first baby the honeymoon is over and the work begins. Not only that, but both parents discover afresh that where two is company three can make for friction. Strong feelings are aroused and old conflicts are relighted. A new equilibrium has to be found.'

Dr Sandra Elliott says, '[Psychiatric] literature has been unusually consistent in finding a relationship between reports of a less than satisfactory marital relationship and postnatal depression,' and lists 14 supporting academic references to be going on with. Dr Jack Dominian says, 'In taking a history of marital difficulties of some standing one of the commonest remarks which is made spontaneously is, "It all started with the birth of Charles/Jenny/Peter . . . and it has been going on ever since." There is little doubt that if all post puerperal disorders were diagnosed in time and both treated and counselled that marital breakdown would become less.'

Finances

Lack of money is a prime source of stress. It is depressing in itself and certainly increases strife. Unemployment has brought an increase in genuine poverty (one in three children in Britain are now growing up in poverty, according to the Maternity Alliance), while the relative decline in income of certain groups and the desire to share in a higher standard of living have combined to make many people feel poorer than they were. Couples who settle down late, or who remarry and want children, find obtaining decent housing is difficult and takes a large portion of their income. Surroundings that are barely noticed by a working couple can turn into a gloomy prison for the mother at home with a little baby.

Managing on one income may seem wellnigh impossible, yet where a woman is modestly paid the cost of childcare can mean it is not worthwhile for her to carry on working, especially with a second or subsequent child. Two financial issues are involved when a mother stops work – reduction in family income and loss of independent income.

An example of the destruction resulting from the loss of an independent income is described by Kay Carmichael in *New Society*. The couple had married young and had a baby early. 'When her pay cheques stopped coming in she asked Douglas how they were going to organise the housekeeping money. Could he give her a monthly cheque? He thought that was a bit silly. It would be simpler just to give her cash every week. That was six months ago. Often he was short and just gave her what he had in his wallet. Now he leaves something every morning. Sometimes he forgets so she has learnt to remind him or she'll be left with nothing.

'She has used up all the savings she had in her own account and she's thinking she'll have to find a childminder job if her self-respect is to survive. Her unthinking love for her husband is corroded with anger at his use of power to humiliate her. He doesn't understand what she is talking about.'

Alternatively, a mother may want to stay at home and be prepared to make financial sacrifices to do so but be pressurised by her partner to return to work 'because we need the money', or feel she ought to contribute in hard cash to the household. The wife of a man who is already supporting a family may be forced to return to work to keep the second family.

A wanted child?

Lack of money can make having a child at all a source of contention between partners. Or it can be used as a cover for avoiding the heavy responsibilities of parenthood. More usually, the woman wants a child while the man is not so sure. If a baby is born in spite of these doubts it can create a big barrier between the couple.

Both partners may be emotionally threatened by the possibility of a child and unable to face the prospect of receiving less attention from each other. An unplanned pregnancy can then precipitate a crisis. Where one partner is emotionally dependent, and does not want to share being loved, they may under pressure appear to give in, agreeing to have a child, but later take it out of their partner as underlying resentment surfaces.

Writing in *Parents* about why men have affairs soon after a baby is born, counsellor Anne Hooper says, 'They restore an emotional balance which may have been lost when the baby became a rival. Men are commonly jealous of their children, sensing – especially with the first one – that the love and attention once directed at them is now being focused on the baby.'

Role divisions

Unless a couple are very self-aware, and regularly discuss their feelings and expectations, the changed priorities and life patterns brought about by having a child can be the source of endless misunderstandings. After the birth the way a couple live out their roles in relation to each other, and their male and female roles in society, is all thrown into question because they are dealing with a new situation. Even if they do not articulate it, women feel that the changes they have made or experience in order to be a mother need to be balanced by changes in the man's life and attitudes, but often he sails on, his life apparently little touched.

Instead of a couple agreeing how their roles will change, they often expect their new life to just shake into place automatically, or women expect their partners to sense telepathically what their new needs are. Where only one partner thinks things through and wants to discuss a different way of running their life but cannot even get the subject discussed, it is usually the woman.

A couple may rub along, without defining or being aware of role divisions, in their relationship or in society generally. But once there is a baby to care for role divisions are thrown sharply into focus. Women may feel distressed because they want to continue as before and cannot, or because they want a change and do not get it. Women who welcomed equality before the birth may want a more traditional division of responsibility once they have a child. They may feel deeply disconcerted if the father impinges on 'their' territory, making decisions about the baby. And many 'liberated' women find themselves feeling disappointed, if not downright cheated, when a man does not expect to keep his wife and children or cannot afford to. A man who has always shared tasks and responsibilities may suddenly cease to do so once there is a child, either as a silent protest at the child's existence, or because he assumes that now his wife does not have a paid job she has enough time to take on everything domestic.

Changing the division of responsibilities and labour within a relationship should only be a pragmatic matter, something that is reviewed automatically whenever work or children alter needs. But changes become very emotionally loaded because the possibility had not been considered, the practical details had not been discussed, one partner does not like the new requirements, or because of underlying insecurities.

Parenting arrangements

Whether the mother does paid work fulltime, part-time or not at all, who does what for the baby is invariably a source of dissension or, where the mother feels childcare is her job regardless of what else she has to do, a source of resentment. Adding to the burden is the dearth of preschool childcare or education facilities, from short session playgroups with mothers in attendance to fulltime day nursery places. In many Continental and Eastern bloc countries 90–95% of three-year-olds receive some professional care outside the home, but elsewhere the expectation is that the mother is the sole carer and is able and willing to stay at home for at least five years.

Ann Oakley slams the usual assumptions about childcare as unrealistic and harmful. In *Radical Science Journal* she says, 'Childcare is gendered work. Our ideas about it are fixed in the aspic of heterosexuality [and] debased Freudian psycho-logic.' And, '. . . maternal depression, paternal distance and child abuse are all unintended but inevitable consequences of current parenting arrangements.'

Individual couples who try to break the mould and share parenting find career structures working against them, especially in the current harsh economic climate. If, in order to be with their children, both parents have breaks in their careers, or forgo seniority by postponing further study or training or deliberately limiting their commitment to work, they may never be allowed back on the ladder, or may be permanently financially disadvantaged. So the woman makes one form of sacrifice by staying at home while her partner makes another by increasing his work load – either to earn more money immediately, or as an investment in his future – when he would rather be more involved in caring for his children. This increases stress on both partners and separates them, depriving them of common ground and of each other's support.

King of the castle

As well as fulltime childcare, most women have another burden they cannot put down – propping up their partners. Whatever problems a man has psychologically or in coping with society's demands, usually he expects his partner to listen to his troubles and to back him, yet he may see her emotional needs as a demand he should not have to meet or does not even want to know about. Whatever frustrations pile up in the outside world, he expects to come in the door and be free to give vent to his anger, and not to be met with any events or attitudes that will increase his sense of being opposed. Mild-mannered male work colleagues can be the most amazing domestic tyrants.

Who cares for the carer? Usually nobody. Indeed, abuse may be her lot. Writing on the hazards of housework, in a Women's Health Information Centre newsletter Lesley Doyal says, 'As well as undertaking the physical labour of "housework" women are also expected to be responsible for childcare. This can obviously be immensely rewarding but many women also find it both physically and emotionally demanding . . . More broadly, women are held responsible for "emotional housework" – managing relationships between the different members of the family and compensating them for their pains and frustrations. Indeed, failure to satisfy what their partners perceive as their needs may even expose women to the most dramatic health hazard of housework – domestic violence.'

Battered women receive few mentions in psychiatric textbooks. The American *Comprehensive Textbook of Psychiatry*, for instance, contains two sentences about domestic violence. Women may well be labelled neurotic or depressed who are actually constantly terrified for their own physical safety or that of their children. Or marital violence can induce neurotic depression in women as a way of coping with emotional deprivation and the ensuing sense of insecurity. Feeling helpless to oppose or escape violence can start in childhood with having a violent or sexually abusing father. And, indeed, there may be no alternative to endurance but living on social security in a women's refuge.

Research suggests that domestic violence is widespread. In their book *Dealing with Depression*, Kathy Nairne and Gerrilyn Smith say of domestic violence, '. . . it is such a private crime. There is enormous pressure on women to maintain the façade of domestic bliss . . . Intermittent or continuous physical violence, often coupled with sexual and mental cruelty, destroys your perception of yourself as a potent capable person. The fact that one person (a male) violates the other (a female) maintains the power imbalances that are present in numerous other forms throughout society . . .

'It is crucial that we recognise the damage physical and sexual violence does to women. If you know no other relationship but an abusive one, it can take a lifetime to recognise and escape from it. The lack of alternatives and support make it very difficult even for the most courageous of us . . .

'Alone and feeling responsible for what has happened to us, we think we are going crazy. This world we live in does not seem as safe. It can become a terrible place to be. We experience a sense of helplessness because violence controls us. Its unpredictability makes it more frightening. These experiences can be surrounded by silence. We frequently don't feel able to tell anyone what happened. When we do, we are not only confronted by disbelief but also a lack of understanding and adequate protection.

'Violence, in any form, penetrates to our very souls. It profoundly affects our sense of self and our estimation of our own worth.'

Sexual problems

Marital conflict often centres on sexual problems, even though these may be only a small part of the total difficulties. Lack of sexual responsiveness by the new mother frequently results from tiredness – she is too weary to be interested in anything. The exhaustion is both physical and emotional. In *Nursing Times* Nurse Kate Ashton says, 'Sexual demands can seem like the last straw to a woman who has been steadily losing sleep and giving out an endless stream of love and attention ever since the birth of her new child. She feels exhausted of love. A conflict emerges within her: who is the most deserving of the finite reserve of love within her? The baby, of course. After all, it won't be forever. The child is helpless. It didn't ask to be born. Her husband agrees wholeheartedly. That does not stop him from wanting and needing his wife. She feels his need. She feels guilty not meeting it.'

The most common and practical reason for a woman not wanting to resume sexual relations soon after her baby is born is that she has had an episiotomy. This cutting of the vaginal entrance may have been badly sited, clumsily done, ill-timed, and sewn up after too long an interval by an inexperienced young doctor. Healing may be poor, the stitches too tight, the scar tissue unyielding.

Physical discomfort or extreme pain on intercourse may persist for months, or even years, and necessitate corrective surgery. In addition to the physical aspects the woman may feel the cut constituted an attack, or some kind of ritual mutilation, especially if she realises that most episiotomies are not necessary (see Chapter 2). The whole birth may have been so physically and pyschologically traumatic that her body and spirit feel bruised and wounded. Or an unpleasant birth may reactivate buried emotions associated with earlier incest, rape or abortion. Once aversion to sex has been established, it is very hard to overcome, and abstinence may become a habit, leading to arguments, affairs and breakdown of the relationship.

But even given good, gentle and intervention free births, it is questionable whether women should be pressurised into feeling it is their duty to be ready and willing to be sexually available soon afterwards, the pressure backed by dire threats of the husband looking elsewhere if he is denied his rights. Some women are filled with sexual desire immediately postnatally and joyfully resume a physical relationship – which may, indeed, have been only briefly interrupted for the birth. Other women, however, feel divided by the demand to return straight away to their sexual role.

A mother's lack of sexual desire when she has had a baby is interpreted only in a negative way as 'loss of libido', 'a sign of depression' and 'psychosexual difficulty', but it can alternatively be viewed as healthy, natural and desirable. Social worker Pauline

Mullins says, 'Childcare begins during the pregnancy when the mother enters a phase known as "primary maternal preoccupation"; the mother dwells on the pregnancy to the exclusion of other interests.' After birth, some women become totally absorbed in the baby – they are 'in love' with it – in a way that makes sex seem irrelevant, and their partners should be able to accommodate and respect this, instead of placing their needs before the baby's in an immature way.

The lack of desire is not a sign that something is wrong, but a temporary sublimation of sexual energy and focus on the partner into protection and nurturance of the tiny baby – it is natural for survival. During this time the mother gets to know her baby and builds an intense bond. If this sense of wonder and protective love temporarily precludes sex, why should a woman have to overcome her instinctive feelings? Why should she have to 'buy' male devotion, fidelity, financial, practical and emotional support for herself and her infant with sex?

There are enormous pressures in magazine articles, from lay organisations and counsellors, and from doctors, psychiatrists and psychotherapists for women to return to being slim, sexy and available soon after having a baby. It is important that women resist these pressures and physical stereotypes. Endlessly trying to alter your image to an imposed notion of beauty is a recipe for mental illhealth. And dieting soon after having a baby can cause exhaustion, physical illhealth and biochemical imbalances. It also interferes with breastfeeding.

Worrying about not being glamorous and about losing your husband, having sex against your wishes, feeling guilty about giving the baby undivided attention, and not eating adequately are all stresses the new mother could do without, and factors likely to harm her physical and emotional health.

FATHERS ARE PEOPLE, TOO

Fathers used to know quite clearly what was expected of them – maintaining the family financially and keeping all its members in line. Today, as writer Maureen Green says, 'The number of men who would now enjoy playing the role of stern Victorian paterfamilias is probably very few . . . They would much prefer being a modern father, if only they could be a little more certain what that is.'

Men and women are very confused as to what they expect, want and need from fatherhood. With no strong guidelines, couples have to make up the role, piecemeal, as they go along. Where a couple are not especially analytical, articulate or communicative about such abstract matters, a gap can easily develop between the woman's ideas and the man's.

There is not much popular material available to men, suggesting what models of fatherhood they could choose from and explaining the conflicts they may feel. They are working in the dark and may desperately need support at a time when they are called on to be supportive of their wife and baby. Yet men are less willing than women to admit to feelings of ambivalence or confusion, to appear at a loss or weak in any way, or to seek help.

Gerry Popplestone, in *MAN* magazine, describes how men learn early to avoid even thinking about anything disturbing. 'Humiliation is a key experience in keeping men in role. The shame of doing something that is considered not masculine is immense. As boys, it is generally so painful for us that we resolve never again to be caught doing something unmasculine. We learn to avoid shame at all costs. It is the shame that keeps us in role. But the skill we pick up is the avoidance tactic: how to avoid any situation where we might be shamed again.'

The other way boys learn not to step out of line is, 'Peer group activity is very strong and teenagers get a lot of support from it. If we fail as kids in our obligation to other kids, we risk rejection. And rejection is a very painful experience. A boy must have mates and every boy soon learns what to do to keep his mates. So we learn to be masculine by avoiding situations where we will feel ashamed or guilty. We don't take risks by acting out of role and we don't let our mates down by showing too much independence. We go along with what is required of us as boys and manage to avoid the painful feelings of guilt and shame.'

It is therefore very hard for a couple to reach an individual balance because they are so programmed and pressured about how they ought to live their life together and deal with birth and children.

Men's involvement in parenthood has increased, with fathers caring for their children in practical ways more often than their fathers did, but a lot of care is optional. Men often choose the more pleasant and sociable tasks, and may make their help conditional on their partner complying with their wishes in other areas. A woman whose partner voluntarily undertakes a lot of childcare and household tasks is seen as unusually lucky. In any case, as several studies and surveys have shown, men's perceptions of how much work they do in the home are generally different to women's – women record their partners' doing a lower percentage of childcare and domestic tasks than the men do.

Sharing the birth

Involvement with their children is seen as stemming from the increased presence of fathers at the births (variously calculated at 70–90%). And being at the birth certainly forges a strong link between some men and their babies, making the child real from the start instead of a funny little stranger. Supporting the mother through the birth brings some partners much closer and increases their respect for each other.

But the experience is very variable. The father may have been ill-prepared for the birth and be quite ignorant of what is happening and so unable to help, or absolutely terrified. He may find the intensity of emotion disturbing and cut off, from it and his partner, or be unable to feel anything. The woman may have ambivalent feelings about her partner that have been well suppressed but surface during labour and birth, or she may prefer a woman's warmth and tenderness. The man then feels angry and shut out. Sometimes surfacing tensions between the couple can interfere with the birth process. Michel Odent says, 'We have noticed that the presence of a man can inhibit the woman and that labour only progressed well after the husband had left the room.'

The main reason that the father's experience of being at the birth is of variable quality is that he is there on tolerance, not of right, unless the couple are in their own home. In hospital, medical authorities *permit* a man to be with his partner. They frequently control the circumstances and amount of contact to such a degree that the link between the couple is fragmented and both are left feeling confused and disappointed. There is no reason to exclude a man while various procedures are carried out. In fact, there is no reason for most of the procedures – which alienate the man from the woman, turning her step by step from his intimate physical partner to a medically controlled object – to be carried out at all.

Permanent damage can be done to the relationship when the man is manipulated into persuading or bullying the woman to accept some intervention she does not want – she may never forgive the betrayal. The doctors usually find the father's co-operation easy to gain. He will probably inherently trust medical science more than his partner, will not have her instinctive faith in the workings of her body, and will be encouraged to see her intense physical efforts as pain from which he ought to rescue her – especially as his action in making her pregnant has 'caused' the pain.

Whatever he was persuaded to believe at antenatal classes about the importance of his role in the birth, the father pretty soon finds that he comes bottom of the pecking order in hospital, and will be shoved firmly back in his place if he has any ideas of his own or tries to put his wife's point of view across. Some more cynical fathers suspect that the reason the medical establishment suddenly caved in on the issue of paternal involvement and now expect a man to stay with his partner during most of labour and birth, is that they realised how useful fathers could be – one as unpaid labour to keep the mother company, run errands, and physically support her, and two as an intermediary in maintaining obstetric control over the mother.

Landing in limbo

While men have been drawn into supervising their partners during labour and rewarded by being allowed to stay for the birth, as soon as they have done their allotted work they are turfed out into the cold. This separation soon after birth causes immense distress for many women who long to cuddle up together as a new family and fall asleep in a warm embrace. But they are settled in a bed, and do have their baby to concentrate on. The man has to walk away from the company, the warmth, the lights, the excitement and drama of the birth, leaving the people he loves the most, to go – usually – to nothing.

Richard Seel points out that the father is left totally in limbo after a hospital birth – there is no formal structure to his life, even his domestic routine has gone. He sees birth as rite of passage that, especially for a man, is missing the final stage of incorporation into society as a new person. Men are left 'up in the air'. They may feel profoundly alienated and even become depressed. Seel thinks that 'At least 90 % of men suffer from some form of depression postpartum.

After the birth, particularly if they have witnessed it, being thrown out is awful.' He believes that even when fathers are not excluded after the birth they still suffer a postpartum sadness, a sense of loss. Some men get 'withdrawal symptoms from the high of it all'. Others unexpectedly find the whole thing very untouching, although they may become devoted fathers.

Seel also says there is a power struggle going on, with great female resistance to males wanting in on birth and childrearing. He is probably right as, for many women, these represent the sole areas within the marriage where they have autonomy and authority and it does not seem likely they will easily be persuaded to share.

Practicalities and realities

At the practical level, couples who do want to share childcare meet problems from the start. Although maternity leave in Britain is still patchy and inadequate, and has received some setbacks, the principal is established. But the great majority of men have no right to paid leave when their children are born. And schemes giving several months' paid or perhaps unpaid leave to either parent, to be taken when desired in the child's early years, are just a dream in Britain, although they have been the subject of a draft EEC directive.

Another problem for fathers is that they are often completely unfamiliar with babies and small children in the flesh, and are not the usual targets of printed or conversational information and advice. Men who wanted to look after their babies may find they do not know how to – they have completely unrealistic expectations of their offspring and find them quite impossible to deal with. Loving the idea of becoming a father, they can find themselves impatient, resentful and even violent towards their children.

Whoever actually does the childcare and increased domestic work, the couple are left with radically less time to be spent exclusively on each other. Babies cannot be rationalised and organised, and a man who is efficient at his job may be perpetually perplexed and frustrated that he cannot reduce the endless hours of fiddling about dealing with a baby entails, and saddened because his old relationship and way of life have vanished in a way he never anticipated. Romance and sex may seem to have gone forever. Richard Seel says, 'Marital satisfaction usually goes plummetting when a baby arrives. There is a great strain on a relationship at the time of birth.'

All the strains and stresses after the birth of a baby may be no worse for men than women, but men tend to have more rigid expectations and find assimilating new experiences harder. Equally, they are more likely to bottle up what they feel, and less likely to make new friends they could share their problems with. Because he is mixed up and unhappy the man will be unable to be supportive to his partner if she is stressed or has developed PND. Or sensing his tension and alienation may actually drive the woman into depression. Either way, they will argue or cease to communicate, according to their temperaments, so increasing their misery and disillusionment.

GOING IT ALONE

'Single parents', 'unmarried mothers' and 'lone parents' are all inaccurate ways of lumping together those women who do not have the support of a fulltime partner in bearing their children, and exclude those women who live with their husbands but find themselves carrying the full burden of parenthood.

Single, widowed or separated mothers may or may not have a fulltime male partner, who may or may not be the father of their baby; they may receive varying degrees of financial support or none at all; they may be sharing their lives with another woman. The woman who is categorised as alone may actually have full support, she may have been deserted partway through her pregnancy or soon after the birth, she may have left the baby's father or her partner, have got pregnant despite knowing she would receive no support, or actually not want to share parenting. A woman may be officially unsupported but have a lot of loving help from family and friends, or be quite alone but financially stable, fully in command of her life and overjoyed to have a child.

The only measure of a mother's loneness is how alone she feels. Given the load they carry, it is remarkable what a good job most lone women make of parenting. Having sole care of a child is unremitting and compounds the problems of exhaustion, isolation and loss of income that most mothers face. For 24 hours a day, seemingly for ever, you are solely responsible for the baby or have to make adequate alternative arrangements for care. Whether exhaustion, isolation or poverty poses the greatest difficulty varies with circumstances and the woman's temperament. The problems are usually inextricably interlinked, making each harder to solve.

Being a lone parent family almost always means being poor, and about 50% of such families are dependent on supplementary benefit. Poverty is probably the single most depressing factor mothers alone face, because it ties their hands in all directions. Without money there is often no way of getting a break from the baby, or even of getting a rest unless the baby sleeps a lot. Mothers who have to take a paid job may find broken nights the last straw, wearing them steadily down through weariness to depression.

Isolation is more difficult to overcome when you are completely broke, especially when this involves being badly housed or homeless. Once childcare costs have eaten into her income, even the working mother may find social activities limited by lack of money. Being busy all day also makes it very difficult to meet other mothers and babies, and women who are alone with children often find themselves excluded from weekend family socialising.

Exhaustion and lack of money often make going out in the evening impossible and, anyway, working mothers see little enough of their babies. Unsupported mothers may be very unhappy at being separated from their child because they are obliged to earn, and strongly resentful of mothers who can stay at home but whine on about how bored they are.

Some women find being a mother, or combining being a mother with a paid job, quite enough to cope with and, looking round the problems their friends have with their partners, are quite glad not to have to fulfill that role as well. However, most women who are alone with a child feel hurt, abandoned and lonely. Women with small children tend to be socially invisible to males, as if they had a 'not available' notice round their necks and thereby ceased to be worth speaking to, but mothers who are alone and reveal that they have no ties are treated warily by men and women alike in case they are looking for someone to rescue them.

Some women really cannot see themselves as complete without a male and are always searching for potential partners. But many women who are alone are not necessarily ready for another relationship, especially if they were badly hurt by the break-up with the baby's father. They do, however, miss attention, physical warmth and a sex life. And they feel the need of someone to discuss things with and share all the responsibilities.

Feeling unlovely and unloved can lead to feeling unloving. The genuinely unsupported mother must be a bottomless well of giving as she is her child's only source of love and reassurance, while she herself is emotionally starving. Staying mentally healthy under these strains is very hard.

Added to this is usually guilt or anger or both at the child's father-less state. With the growing number of irregular family set-ups and children born outside wedlock the social stigma of illegitimacy has decreased, and the legal status is being abolished, but the practical disadvantages of not having a good father are obvious, while the enormous emotional deprivation probably cannot be compensated for. Feeling emotional pain herself, the mother who is alone is only too aware of the heritage of pain passed to her baby. But because there is no one to share her responsibilities she will have to bury her disturbance deep in order to carry on functioning, even if in a damaged fashion. Her distress becomes like a time bomb, sure to go off at some stage, uncertain in what havoc that will cause.

GROWING UP

Becoming a mother both requires and stimulates personal growth. It is a maturational event, extending from the time when the mother realises she wants to conceive to the time when she is happy to define herself as a mother, having integrated and harmonised the elements of her old and new selves.

Having a baby forces women to grow up, however unevenly and incompletely, overnight. Clearly the more growing up that was done before the birth – getting to know, like and respect herself, clearing out emotional cupboards, realising what she needs from her partner and what price she is prepared to pay to have her needs met, under-standing why she wants to be pregnant and have child – the easier her transition to motherhood will be.

It is necessarily a period of adjusting to losses and assimilating gains, a period of destabilisation when everything is thrown into the melting pot in order for a new identity to be forged. The further along the path a woman has gone before her pregnancy, the less likely she is to completely lose her balance. Attaining motherhood will be a maturational progression, not a crisis (see Chapter 7).

Why children?

One measure of being grown up is whether a woman is able to work out clearly why she wanted to be pregnant, and what she expects from the child. Sometimes women want their lives to be more exciting and have a secret desire to be swept along by events stronger than themselves, to dice with the forces of life and death. When they find they are actually pregnant they may be horrified. Or they may crave the warm, full feeling of being pregnant, but not actually want to give birth or be responsible for a child. They may want a baby to change their lives or give them status – not for itself. If they yearn for love and physical affection, they may want a child, believing they will give it love but actually expecting the baby to love them. Most women's motives for getting pregnant are mixed and that will not necessarily cause a woman problems if she recognises what they are and does not believe the baby can supply her needs.

Struggling to awareness

There is a lot working against the woman who wishes to grow up. Growing up implies assuming responsibility for oneself, and women are taught to leave responsibility for themselves in other people's hands – first their parents and teachers, then their partners, bosses, doctors, lawyers, anyone who represents authority and the state. Women have internalised their inadequacy and unworthiness for too long for it to be easy for individuals to overcome in their own life-times. Fortunately, that does not stop a lot of women trying, but what should be a natural flowering often turns into a stressful, depressing battle.

The male condition is taken to be the human condition, men are an embodiment of the norm. Women are not men, so they are not the norm (or normal?), are inherently lacking, deficient, inferior. They are seen as subjective not objective, and therefore unreliable. They are not fit to be in charge of their persons and their lives. Women learn to fear stepping out of line and police their own behaviour. A woman who does not conform is seen as unhealthy, in need of shepherding back into the fold. Worse, she may merely become invisible. Her opinion is not even worth countering. Standing out in the cold, deprived of the usual rewards of being conventionally feminine, she is likely to give up and step back inside. By the time she has discovered the rewards are illusory, it is even harder for her to go her own way.

Growing up successfully is made more difficult because it is hard for women to know or understand themselves, or pin down why they feel ill at ease with their role. This is because, as feminist Andrea Dworkin says, 'We live in a male-imagined world, and our lives are circumscribed by the limits of male imagination. Those limits are very severe.' For women there is a great disjunction between what they are told they will feel and will make them happy and what actually happens, but they are hampered in analysing this situation by lack of female-defined concepts and language. Nor are women offered a variety of healthy models of thinking and feeling. Instead they are likely to be encouraged to do a footbinding job on their feelings and potential. Neatly crippled, they are not in a position to give much trouble. Many women cannot envisage themselves as self-contained, self-regulating, confident, mature, 'grounded' people, or reconcile these qualities with being accepted as feminine. They do not manage to grow up before they become pregnant, when mother-hood catches them short, in urgent need of mothering themselves.

In need of mothering

However mature a woman is, the transition to motherhood is made easier by support from a maternal figure, someone who has been there already and can be tender, sympathetic and nurturant without taking over the mother or failing to exercise respect for her authority and decision making. And even the most 'together' woman can find the drama of birth brings unrecognised skeletons out of the cup-board, suddenly creating an intense need for support from a strong, uncritical woman.

Where a woman has no mother, or a poor relationship with her, during the birth and afterwards she may seek maternal qualities in her partner who may be quite unable to answer her dependency needs. The confusion that occurs if a man is called on to support his partner when a child arrives is compounded if he considers her to be his surrogate mother. He is being called on to mother his mother, while being displaced as her child.

A woman may acknowledge that her lover is also a friend, perhaps

a 'brother'. She may realise that he is also a son figure, or that he con-
nives in postponing her full maturation by being a father figure. But it is
rare for a couple to be consciously aware of and openly acknowledge
the inherent contradictions and stresses of a lover being required to
supply a mother's missing nurturance. The situation becomes increasingly unhealthy and dangerous where an immature woman who
craves mothering but has been called on to do a lot of emotional housework for her partner builds up a backlog of need before she has a baby.
Once she has a child she has no resources with which to meet its needs.

Because of their economic or social situation or a poor relationship,
emotionally, intellectually and sensually many women are on a starvation diet after birth. If they have rich reserves these will probably see
them through. But some women have not been nurtured or mothered
since babyhood, or perhaps never at all. When they are suddenly
called on to put out to the baby ceaselessly, this precipitates a crisis.
They may become completely numb or break down, overwhelmed by
the pain of their unmet needs.

Various studies have revealed that many depressed mothers report
unhappy childhoods, with disturbed parents. Unresolved conflicts
between a woman and her parents will hinder her development and
are likely to resurface at times of stress. For a woman, becoming a
parent herself is peculiarly potent in stirring up unfinished business.
Sometimes the resulting crisis enables mother and daughter to heal
old wounds, but often the daughter seeks a new relationship based on
an increased understanding of her mother's own difficulties in being a
parent, only to be further wounded by the older woman's refusal to
open up or come to meet her. The older mother may just not want to
have her emotions disturbed, or she may resent her daughter in a
variety of ways and take this opportunity of hurting and punishing her.

Taking charge

Women are more vulnerable to being hurt by their partners because
they are brought up to place themselves in others' hands, to pass themselves over for safekeeping. They may come to realise the folly of this,
yet be unable to break the habit, because they need a man to give them
affirmation of self – Prince Charming is the source of everything for
them.

Sheila Kitzinger regards romance as dangerous because (like

pornography) it does not treat sex realistically nor acknowledge a woman as a person. In *Cosmopolitan* she says romance 'distorts everything that is real in human experience and snuffs out a girl's potential to be herself and do what she wants. Self-worth becomes something that is conferred on a woman by a man and lasts only as long as he wants her.'

When the dream fails, women see themselves as prisoners, helpless to make their own happiness. In *You* Irma Kurtz records Mai Zetterling's view of her adolescent self as 'already locked into the bitterness that holds so many women captive . . . so they spend a lifetime blaming and despairing, waiting to be rescued.' Mai Zetterling saw the light and broke out, but many women find growing up and taking charge of their lives too uncomfortable or difficult without assistance that is usually lacking.

A period of independence, whether spent at work, in training or education, hopefully can provide an opportunity for the personality to grow, for girls to have a chance to become individuals, with wider horizons and greater resources, before becoming mothers. However, education is not neutral and girls absorb attitudes and expectations along with facts and skills. Their education may still encourage them to limit their growth and responsibility for self in certain ways.

Women can lock themselves into their roles, fearing change. When their partner wants to help with the baby and the housework, they feel undermined and threatened and cling to the status quo while resenting the extra work they have to do. Mental and emotional rigidity, together with lack of confidence, prevents them from sharing the area they do control. They will not allow themselves or their relationship to grow.

In addition, where women have a good enough job to live independently before they set up home with a man they may appear and believe themselves to be sophisticated and adult, but the demands of motherhood can reveal a mass of unresolved emotional conflict and dependency needs which have blocked their path to maturity.

Self-fulfilment

The ideology of 'the rights of the individual' has led to a quest for personal fulfilment and self-realisation, and relationships with lovers are seen to be desirable and workable only in as much as they further that aim. Personal fulfilment is a productive aim, but viewing one's partner as a means to achieving that state imposes a severe if not impossible burden on a relationship.

Once a baby arrives the practical barriers to pursuing self-fulfilment are enormous, and any attempts may have to be accepted as unrealistic for several years. It is a great shock for many women to realise, as it happens to them, the enormous hidden impoverishment of women's lives that motherhood entails, often concealed by a relatively high standard of living for the whole family. Most mothers have little or no time, money or space to call their own, and to someone immature this deprivation may be intolerable and lead to terrific outbursts of violence or apathy plus quiet desperation. Pressure to 'keep up with things', stay glamorous and be sociable just fuels the problem, making the mother feel frustrated and a failure as she contemplates the impossible.

'Postponement of gratification' sounds unwelcomely Victorian but may be the only realistic course to adopt, given the inflexible circumstances in which many mothers find themselves. However, this lack of opportunity for personal realisation makes it all the more important to have grown up as much as possible before this period. The switch to growing through giving may be quite impossible for someone who has not reached a reasonable level of development, and the need for a mother to act maturely and unselfishly, to sustain a helpless new being, combined with lack of opportunity to find and digest the cultural and social food needed for mental growth, may lead to a complete breakdown.

One mother described the enormous drain on her resources after the birth of her triplets. 'Any postpartum depression I might have suffered was indistinguishable from the general struggle of being overwhelmed ... Over a period of time I noticed that my mind suffered ... It was like becoming senile. All of my psychic energy was going into sustaining the babies and the family.' (Boston *Our Bodies, Ourselves*) While her circumstances were peculiarly demanding, it is typical that she received little support and had to delve deep into herself to survive. Women definitely need practical and emotional support after the birth if they are not to break down or strain their mental and physical resources, laying the ground for future trouble. Yet many women have no one to help them, or are too immature and insecure to be willing to accept what help is offered.

96

POWER AND ANGER

Whatever the way in which a disturbed woman is manifesting her distress, talking with her will almost always reveal that she is actually angry, sometimes about everything in her life. She is angry because she lacks power – it is not even left to her to define who and what she is. This fierce, consuming anger has to be considered socially because it results from a lack of control which is socially and politically determined. Women cannot control the way they give birth, their finances, housing and general living conditions, the male/female power balance, or the conditioning to which they are subjected and the expectations they are supposed to meet.

Of course, social circumstances and expectations limit men's lives and are often beyond their control. But however low down the power ladder they are, they invariably feel superior to women as a class and their female partner in particular – hardly surprising as everything in society re-inforces that view. It is only surprising that some men are immune to this conditioning or make great efforts to overcome it, as this can demand much self-sacrifice and leave them in a no-man's land. Many young male hopefuls give up and settle into middle-aged domestic tyranny, or find their 'true' attitudes surfacing once their partner is pregnant. Having the financial whiphand encourages assumption then abuse of power.

Women feel both angry and powerless because of the contradictions built into their life plans – contradictions which become particularly visible when women become mothers. A London Women and Mental Health Group broadsheet describes this situation. 'From birth our lives are shaped by messages about what we are allowed to be and how we should behave as female children and women. The images of women endlessly pasted up and churned out by the media tell that "normal" women are gentle, passive and available at all times, as seductive partners for men, and as cooks, cleaners and nurses for the whole family. The experience of our mothers and other women show us how to play this role, and at the same time, how impossible it is to become the ideal woman. Despite the fact that the realities of most women's lives do not match this ideal, and that some women's hopes and dreams contradict it, it is still the standard by which we are judged . . .

'To survive as "normal" "feminine" women, we have to repress so much of ourselves – our assertiveness, feelings of competition, desire to be powerful, to think intelligently, to explore and express our sexuality. In turn we also repress our anger at having to deny these parts of ourselves . . . When women show their anger, they are more likely to be thought of as "mad" than "bad".'

Power always equates with masculine, and women who openly exercise power are seen as unfeminine. Even the gentler traits of a 'truly masculine man' are the result of having a position of power. You can be chivalrous, protective, supportive and so on only if you are more powerful than the person you have decided to be nice to. Men have more choices. To be able to choose is to have power. An out-of-work man feels emasculated because many of his choices have gone and he has lost power, and it is thought quite proper for him to be angry. But 'feminine' women are not allowed to show they are angry. Women have internalised this prohibition on protest so deeply that they feel they have no right to be angry, no matter what is done to them or how much they are excluded from the ranks of the fully human. They may not even realise they are angry, until careful questioning begins to take the lid off the cauldron.

Male-defined everything and male language produce a wordless, nameless, nebulous, unfocused discomfort with what is happening which makes repression of feeling almost inevitable. If you cannot work out what is going on, formulate it for yourself, communicate it to those around you, put your point of view to the world at large, and get a favourable reaction, somewhere along the line you will give up and push the uncomfortable thoughts down. The effort involved in trying to formulate something not usually defined causes stress and anxiety. Further anxiety is felt when a woman makes progress in understanding what is happening – what 'they' are doing to her – and begins to register what the implications of seeing this thing through would be. Just as she is starting to get angry, survival demands that she buries everything deep. To be openly angry is to risk social condemnation. To protest is also to risk losing the support of a male partner, especially financially. For the pregnant woman or new mother this is a dangerous or impossible course. Financial power is still mostly in male hands and few women can support themselves and their children in comfort.

Birth is such a major life event that all kinds of hidden feelings tend to be stirred up. In addition, the position of women in general may come sharply into focus for the first time. The birth itself may have demonstrated to a woman her powerlessness. If things are not going the way a woman wants in labour, the worst thing she can do is be polite about it, yet she will feel she ought to be. She has a right to be angry and to express that anger in an effort to change what is happening. But, through biochemical changes, her anger may slow or stop the birth process, as can the conflict of repressing that anger, bringing further obstetric interventions.

If a woman was swept through labour by others' decisions and realises straight afterwards she is angry, it is healthier to be vocal about this, or at least to pour out the feelings on paper with a view to writing a cool letter later. 'If you don't express your anger, you could end up depressed. And your anger is justified,' says Margaret Wright, an activist working in the home birth movement. But often women do not realise they are angry, only that they are miserable after what should have been a wonderful event.

This anger and general mixed emotions after birth can remain 'unfinished business', festering away, because women have so little time and energy to devote to themselves once there is a baby to care for. They do not have opportunities to think through what has happened or make connections between the birth and how they feel now, so they stay namelessly deeply angry. The anger can be driven back in to become self-destruction – suicidal depression.

The destructive emotion that patriarchally educated 'mind specialists' see in the new mother as guilt and self-doubt is often the repressed stirrings of anger. Freudians' 'unfocused anxiety' of early childhood origin could well be 'unfocused anger', dating from childhood and rekindled by the birth, the realities of being a mother, new awareness of a partner's attitudes, which all add up to a realisation of powerlessness and a sense of being trapped and oppressed. Deep feelings of worthlessness and inadequacy postnatally are professionally regarded as a manifestation of mental disturbance or sickness. But they may be an accurate reflection of how the mother feels male-dominated society views her. She reasons that if she has been allocated no power she must be of very little value.

Some women absorb male logic and use it to make a protected space for themselves. As women are 'weaker' it is half-expected that they will fall victim to physical and mental ill health, and some women may choose to become ill, or at least not fight unwellness too hard. Even if it makes their state worse in the long run, because they have fulfilled expectations and provided evidence that women are second class, it is inevitable that women (like any other group with limited power) will use what weapons they have. If a woman becomes delicate, weak, out of sorts, or physically or mentally downright ill, she cannot be expected to do too much, and has achieved agreement that it is impossible for her to 'pull herself together'. As long as she can function enough to scrape through her domestic chores she will be left alone. Especially, she can opt out of sex. However limited or negative it is, she has developed a way of asserting herself, of holding out against the male – individual or as a class.

Powerlessness and repressed anger can wreak havoc with a woman's mental and physical health. The physical symptoms of the resulting depression are not imagined or self-induced, but real and produced by biochemical changes. Variable, elusive and low grade, they cause steady attrition of the spirit and willpower. As with the similar symptoms of viral infections such as glandular fever, because nothing dramatic or visible occurs the sufferer is accused of being selfpitying, whining, feeble-spirited and malingering. Ignored medically, the depressed woman begins to doubt her own judgement, be guilty about asking for help, and so become further isolated in her mental distress. Again, lack of relevant language and concepts may make her powerless to voice her inner conviction that she is not mad but physically ill.

The new mother's biochemical functioning is in a period of transition and adjustment, so vulnerable. Once any number of social stresses have interfered with its return to normal, and she feels depressed, the downward spiral starts, because everything is then seen though grey spectacles, perhaps in marked contrast to the rose-hued ones she wore when pregnant. Because all elements of her life seem so depressing they do depress her further.

Because birth brings many changes the mother can become so disorientated that she does not know which part of her life or role represents the 'real' her. Lacking a baseline, she cannot then make meaningful, valid, useful decisions about further changes and action that would improve her life. Even if she can work out what is bothering her and causing disturbed feelings, she may then find most of it is outside her control to alter and improve. Especially when deep exhaustion has set in, she may feel totally powerless to find happiness again.

Chapter 4

Not all in the mind

A variety of psychosocial factors and the type of birth a woman has increase the stresses on her system around the time her baby is born (see Chapters 3 and 2). These stresses can disrupt biochemical functioning to produce depression and emotional and mental disturbances postnatally. Some women inherit abnormalities of biochemical functioning that make them particularly susceptible to PND when they are stressed after birth.

Certain doctors and health workers believe biochemical imbalances are unavoidable and that nothing much can be done to prevent or treat them. Others assume mental distress has no physical causes and direct attention solely to psychotherapeutic solutions (see Chapter 5). Psychiatrists agree that changes in mood and behaviour are accompanied by chemical changes in the body and brain, though there is disagreement as to what is cause and effect. Many psychiatrists and GPs seek to reverse these changes by the administration of drugs. Stresses on a pregnant woman are of many kinds – spiritual, emotional, mental, physical, nutritional, environmental. Yet making a concerted effort to reduce pressures from all sources while at the same time fortifying women's bodies to deal with unavoidable stress without malfunctioning (discussed in this chapter) is rarely considered as an option.

Once a woman has PND, when drugs are used to treat the condition prescribing is not usually preceded by any blood or tissue tests, doses may be massive, the choice of drug haphazard and experimental, and the period of prescription absurd. The immoderate treatment afforded to one woman who became depressed after the birth of her third child, and remained severely disturbed for seven years, is described by psychiatrist Dr Richard Mackarness in *Not All In The Mind*. 'The variety and quantity of medication she was on was prodigious even by psychiatric standards: 25mg of imipramine (Tofranil) three times a day, plus 50mg of trimipramine (Surmontil) at night (these two are powerful antidepressants), and 5mg of haloperiodol (Seranace) three times a day [a major tranquilliser] . . . She was also given 100mg of orphenadrine (Disipal) three times a day to counter-act the haloperiodol's side-effects – muscular rigidity, tremors and excessive salivation.

'At night she got 10mg of nitrazepam (Mogadon), a sleeping pill, and she was down for injections of 10mg of haloperiodol and 10mg of procyclidine (Kemadrin) as necessary to control her outbursts of slashing and running away. On top of all this, she was getting a tablet of fenfluramine (Ponderax) twice a day for her obesity, and a daily Norinyl contraceptive pill lest she become pregnant – not that she had much sex drive under all this medication and depression, but the policy was "better safe than sorry".' Electroconvulsive therapy had been added, for good measure. She had been variously diagnosed as having 'schizophrenia, schizo-affective psychosis, presenile dementia, temporal lobe epilepsy, neurotic depression and anxiety hysteria.' She was recommended to have surgery on the brain (leucotomy, now in disrepute) that would have permanently altered her personality.

Yet, while willing to use drastic chemotherapy that may produce no improvements but does have major side-effects, psychiatrists invariably dismiss the idea of dealing biochemically with mood dis-turbances, let alone severe mental illness, in more subtle, discrete and accurately targeted ways. In ways that help the body to help itself. Some such approaches are hormone treatments, change of diet, nutritional supplementation, or tracking down and removing foods and environmental substances to which the body is reacting adversely. For example, when Dr Mackarness was allowed a chance to help the woman mentioned above, he decided she was a particu-larly severe case of food allergy. After his treatment she was discharged home on no medication at all.

For women who have PND, psychiatrists' disagreements as to whether altered states of mind follow changes in brain chemistry or cause them are an academic luxury. Of course, ongoing dedicated research to increase all aspects of understanding of mental distur-bances and illness is necessary in order to find new and better treatments, to refine those that do exist, and to eliminate those that are found to have dangers or be counterproductive. But what moth-ers need is help, now. Action may be literally lifesaving.

A lot is already known about changing mood through the use of hormones and nutritional substances and by eliminating allergens, even if it is not always known in exactly what way these measures work. If treatment which is limited to the use of naturally occurring substances in the form, combination and quantities in which they are usually required by the body, or the avoidance of substances that cause an individual to react adversely, is effective, is it not better for women with PND to be offered now what is available and relatively safe, following up precisely how it works when there is time and money available?

Non-drug biochemical ways of treating or preventing PND work by mimicking and aiding the body's own self-balancing mechanisms, and the more any treatment does this the safer and more efficient the process must be. Synthesised wonder drugs, especially in large doses, and ECT hardly parallel ways in which the body tries to achieve homoeostasis. Antidepressant drugs (see Chapter 5) may remove the symptoms of depression but they cannot touch its original causes, emotional or physical. When they do act effectively it is at the cost of a list of side-effects.

Earl Mindell and William H Lee, both American pharmacists and nutritionists, say, 'Drug interactions are so complicated and confusing and hidden that a computer would be hard put to answer every doubtful combination.' They list possible problems as 'drug-food reactions, drug-drug reactions, drug-malnutrition reactions, drug-nutrition reactions; and there are individual drug allergies and idiosyncrasies.'

In discussing the psychological symptoms of allergy sufferers, consultant allergist Dr L M McEwan says, 'it is common to experience long periods of extreme mental fatigue'. He goes on, 'Unfortunately, classical psychiatrists put the cart before the horse; they assume that brain fag is a consequence of "depression". This confusion is a pity because brain fag is not depression and does not respond to anti-depressive drugs.'

ECT and drug treatments try to take short cuts. It is also assumed that the greater the biochemical imbalance the more powerful must be the drug prescribed, the higher the dose, the longer the time it must be given. On the contrary, the greater the imbalance, the more damaging extreme intervention will be. A system that is slightly malfunctioning is still capable of righting itself – and probably would do so quite adequately if either left alone or given minimal help. It is

103

still capable of achieving homoeostasis – maybe even if it is ill-treated, for example with mindbending drugs. On the other hand, one that is expressing its distresss by exhibiting severe and dramatic symptoms is liable to be blasted equally out of balance, but in another direction, or temporarily cease functioning, or always there-after malfunction, if heavyhanded, clumsy intervention is used.

Non-drug biochemical ways of treating PND offer other bonuses. Antidepressants are slow to act, improvements being measured over weeks rather than days, but mood changes induced by including in or excluding from the diet different foods or micronutrients can happen in two or three days, or even hours. And it is certainly easier to control what goes in our mouths than change society overnight – economically, politically, socially, or in terms of male-female rela-tionships. That is not, of course, any reason to stop trying to bring about changes. However, she who survives lives to fight another day: if you are suffering from PND, you are not in a fit state to go out campaigning.

HORMONAL FACTORS

The hormonal changes that occur during pregnancy and at birth are unique in their magnitude and rapidity. Following birth the bio-chemical variation that receives most attention is the drop in oestrogen and progesterone output. Whether the extremely low levels of these sex hormones and imbalances between them are actually abnormal and whether these changes cause the symptoms of PND is the subject of much controversy. Some authorities believe that other hormonal variations are also involved in producing the symptoms of PND, so postnatal hormonal problems are considered to have a variety of causes and possible treatments. The most direct way used of trying to right the balance is by adminstering progesterone itself.

It is usually accepted that the brief 'blues' close after birth are caused by sudden fluctuations in hormonal levels. Because for many women the blues are transient, little medical attention is given to their prevention or alleviation, although there may be many ways of helping or inducing the body to get through this time satisfactorily. This cavalier approach is not good enough. Even if the blues are brief, 50–70% of new mothers are affected so the sum total of hours of misery is high. In addition, the later-occurring severe puerperal psychosis, which has a dramatic onset, is likely to be hormonally caused and therefore avoidable or reversible by influencing hormonal levels. The blues may be an indicator of vulnerability to puerperal psychosis and, for that reason, too, should be accorded greater attention. Non-psychotic postnatal depression has some characteristics which are not usually found in typical clinical depression. Dr Katharina Dalton lists irritability, a never satisfied yearning for sleep, relative alertness in the morning, hunger and thirst. She says 'postnatal depression is atypical because it can only start after pregnancy' and considers there is a hormonal involvement here, too.

Dr Dalton is the person who has done most to pioneer an understanding of the emotional and mental effects on women of certain hormonal changes, and to try to produce an effective answer. A GP and gynaecological endocrinologist best known for her work on premenstrual syndrome or tension, she has fought for over 30 years for an acceptance that women need and deserve sympathetic understanding, accurate diagnosis and swift treatment for premenstrual syndrome and postnatal depression, which she sees as linked.

Her methods of testing her theories and the treatments she uses have been greeted by some other medical people with everything from reservation to total scepticism. As research continues to produce a greater understanding of hormones and related substances, rather than directly administering progesterone as Dr Dalton does, it may prove more effective to prescribe other hormones or to treat and prevent PND through diet and nutritional supplements that affect hormonal levels. But Dr Dalton must be given credit for the discoveries she has made, for caring enough about women's distress to do something, for her tireless devotion to her cause, and for her willingness to help mothers or other doctors who approach her (see Getting Help). The women she has treated successfully think the world of her, feel they can trust their judgement of her work, and continue to spread her ideas enthusiastically.

Dr Dalton firmly believes that PND is different from other forms of depression in several ways (see Chapter 1). She also says, 'There is inevitable confusion with the words "depression" for this suggests that it is all in the mind, whereas to the sufferer it's all in the body . . . It is an illness due to a biochemical abnormality in the brain, which controls the workings of the body, and also a biochemical abnormality in the blood which perfuses all the tissues of the body.' (*Depression After Childbirth*)

Freud, always thought to be on the side of those who oppose hormonal causes and treatments of depression, foresaw the potentialities of biochemistry. In 1927 he said, 'I am firmly convinced that one day all of these disturbances we are trying to understand will be treated by means of hormones or other substances.'

Dalton's theories and methods

Hormones are chemical substances manufactured in one organ, an endocrine gland, and circulated in the blood to act in a specific and limited way on another organ or organs, usually some distance away. Minute quantities produce profound effects, but hormones are only able to work if the biochemical conditions are exactly right.

Hormones, principally oestrogen and progesterone, control menstruation, pregnancy and birth. The pituitary is one of the glands making hormones that govern reproductive changes. It is attached to and interacts with the hypothalamus at the base of the brain. The hypothalamus is a nervous centre which, amongst other vital functions, is involved in the regulation of menstruation, says Dr Dalton. It is 'also the controlling centre for mood, sleep, weight and day/night rhythm . . . during postnatal depression the mood, sleep, weight and day/night rhythms are disturbed.'

The levels of the various menstrual hormones vary throughout the cycle. Progesterone is scarcely present during the first part of the cycle, but increases at ovulation, peaks, then declines to minuscule levels again at menstruation. If there is a deficiency of progesterone, relative to the amount of oestrogen present, premenstrual syndrome with its unpleasant physical and mental symptoms can occur.

Within hours of conception the fertilised egg affects a woman's hormones. During pregnancy hormonal levels rise dramatically and some other hormones, not present at any other time, will be produced. Oestrogen and progesterone rise throughout this time, produced first by the ovaries, later by the placenta. Towards the end of pregnancy progesterone levels are 30–50 times the average peak levels in the menstrual cycle. Another hormone that reaches high levels in pregnancy is prolactin, produced by the pituitary, which prepares the breasts for lactation.

At birth hormonal output changes dramatically. Some hormones cease being made, others are reduced suddenly and their ratios change. Prolactin continues to be produced in large quantities, for breastfeeding. Oestrogen levels in the blood are about 100 times less by day 3 after the birth than in pregnancy and halve again by day 7, remaining level until the menstrual cycle starts up again. Progesterone is some 21 times less by day 3, and disappears by day 7.

Hormones affect mood, and lack of progesterone, or low levels in relation to oestrogen, can produce any of these symptoms: anxiety, irritability, mood swings, nervous tension, aggression; fatigue, lethargy; depression, forgetfulness, crying, confusion, insomnia, low sex drive. Dr Dalton believes that some women's bodies find difficulty in adjusting to this sudden loss, and later in re-establishing an even pattern within the menstrual cycle, so they suffer from PND, and usually PMS when menstruation resumes.

It has never been explained why these women are so sensitive to a sudden fall in progesterone postnatally when, in terms of survival of the species, their bodies should be programmed to adapt. One reason may be that the hypothalamus, at this time, is taking a hammering in all directions. It controls many functions (see earlier), including water balance, hunger and body temperature. During labour and birth, then postnatally because of dealing with the baby's needs, sleep and day/night rhythms are interrupted and disrupted. Then the excessive heat in hospital wards, plus hospital food followed by snatched, irregular meals at home further hamper this nervous centre's attempts to restore to normal everything it regulates. Interventions in the birth, including the administration of hormones, further confuse the issue (see Chapter 2).

In Dr Dalton's studies of the susceptibility of women to PND she has ruled out several factors which might be thought to predispose mothers to PND. She has found no past psychiatric histories in mothers who respond to progesterone therapy. But there does seem to be a genetic element involved. – having a mother or identical twin who has had PND is a risk factor. She has also found that among mothers who had mild depression that required medical help with one pregnancy, 58% developed PND after subsequent births. Of those who had puerperal psychosis, 84% became depressed after another birth. And women who have very high levels of progesterone during pregnancy, and experience a great feeling of well-being, seem especially susceptible to depression, presumably because the change in progesterone is particularly marked for them.

Dr Dalton has been using progesterone to treat PND for some 15 years, and has gradually standardised the regime she uses. She recommends 100mg progesterone, injected intramuscularly after labour and daily for seven days, followed by progesterone suppositories for two months or until the return of menstruation. Progesterone cannot be taken orally because, as it passes through the digestive system, it is deactivated by the liver.

In a recent study, using this regime to prevent the recurrence of PND in women who had received medical treatment for it after previous pregnancies, the recurrence rate was 10%. This compares with another group of women who had experienced PND previously but went untreated in a subsequent pregnancy and had a recurrence rate of 68%. In view of these results, and the numbers of women in PND support groups who say they have been helped, it is hard to see why doctors are so resistant to the implications of Dr Dalton's work.

Critics have said that no-one has consistently demonstrated endocrine differences between women who are depressed and those who are not, and that many women do not improve when given hormones. On the latter point, some women have been given the synthetic hormone progestogen, which can make symptoms worse by lowering the blood level of progesterone. And progesterone needs to be given in time to prevent depression becoming established: it is not claimed to be a cure.

While enormous technical advances have been made in methods of ascertaining hormonal levels it is still true that medical understanding of the way they work and the chemistry of the brain are limited and that, as Dr Dalton says, knowledge 'relies on measurements of hormones in the blood of the body, as opposed to the blood which crosses the blood-brain barrier and bathes the tissues of the brain, or the levels of hormones within the cells of the brain.'

Our knowledge of what is normal in female hormonal levels is limited, too. Dr Guy Abraham, former professor of obstetrics and gynaecology at the University of Calfornia, Los Angeles, is a tireless researcher into female hormones. Trying to establish a baseline for what is normal, it took him three years to find 14 women who were totally free of PMS symptoms or factors that would affect hormonal levels, such as being on the pill.

If the case isn't proven to everyone's satisfaction for the role of hormones in PND, it certainly is not proven against either. Only more research can clarify the matter.

Premenstrual syndrome

There seems to be an overlap between PMS and PND. It has been found that 56% of PMS sufferers who have children will get PND. And many women first get PMS after having a baby. Four or five PMS sufferers out of 10 are short of progesterone, a few women have too much oestrogen, and one in 20 has too much prolactin. As PMS is indisputably hormonally linked, this is further evidence that PND has a hormonal basis.

The key symptoms of tiredness, irritability and depression, exhibited in many postnatal disturbances, are the same as those prevalent in premenstrual tension (part of PMS). And indeed, consultant psychiatrist Dr Diana Riley found that PMS sufferers had a higher incidence of severe depression both on day 5 (23% as against 3%) and one year (20% as against 5%) after the birth. In her study the maternity blues occurred only in those women who reported having suffered from PMS. As it is thought that 30–40% of women of child-bearing age may suffer significant PMS, there must be a lot of women at risk, and so, potentially, a lot of women who could be helped to avoid PND.

Considering PMS after birth, Dr Dalton says that 85% of women who have PND symptoms severe enough to warrant medical help, later, as their PND disappears, start to suffer from PMS. She is concerned that what is regarded as persistent, intractable PND may actually be PMS which could respond to progesterone therapy.

Eating the placenta

Many people have noted that animals eat the hormone-rich placenta after birth, but Dr Dalton states that, 'that cannot be to overcome the rapid drop in hormone levels as the hormones would be broken down by digestion and would be unlikely to be absorbed.' However, midwife Mary Field suffered postpartum psychosis after the birth of her first child and wanted to protect herself against a repeat. As well as ensuring she had a completely different birth at home, she overcame the taboos surrounding human placenta eating.

Swallowing small raw sections of her baby's placenta warded off PND as far as she is concerned. 'Postnatal euphoria set in – I was strong and felt I could do anything . . . Every time I felt tearful I ate a small chunk of raw placenta and found it to be an instant anti-depressant.' She attributes her strength to the steroids in the placenta as these hormones have a powerful body-building effect. Other signs that the hormones were being absorbed by her system were that her milk supply was abundant on day 2, bleeding lasted for only 10 days (it had been 5 weeks with the first baby), and her skin and hair, which the first time had become dry and coarse after the birth, both stayed smooth and silky – 'I retained the bloom of pregnancy'. The placenta is also rich in zinc (see later) and iron.

Possibly, as with many chemicals, the body will absorb and utilise them in their naturally occurring form, in the presence of other substances, some of which have never been identified, whereas it cannot benefit in the same way from an isolated, extracted item, let alone a synthesised one. As it is unlikely that many women will stomach raw placenta, perhaps new mothers should donate their placentas for freeze drying, to be used by other women in tablet or powder form.

Breastfeeding

The question as to whether or not breastfeeding mothers stand a greater chance of getting PND or are protected from it, while breast-feeding or when stopping, has not been clearly answered yet.

Milk production and the adaptation of the breast for feeding are governed by hormones. Prolactin levels, which are high in preg-nancy, continue so for 2–8 weeks after the birth if the mother does not breastfeed. If she breastfeeds, as long as her baby suckles fre-quently and for reasonable periods, prolactin levels stay high.

Dr Dalton has found that some women with PND have milk in their breasts two or three months after stopping breastfeeding, and she has treated them with the drug bromocriptine. Bromocriptine is an ergot derivative which lowers the level of prolactin and hastens the return of ovulation and menstruation, and so normal levels of progesterone.

An extreme example of the apparent link between prolactin and depression occurred in one woman who had very high prolactin levels that required treatment before she could get pregnant. Ten days after her baby was born she stopped breastfeeding. By a month after the birth she had severe PND. Her prolactin levels were found to be 28 times normal and she was prescribed bromocriptine. After 10 weeks on this, she felt her normal self again.

Three psychiatrists in New Zealand suggested that weaning could be a causative factor in psychiatric disturbances after observing a patient who had two episodes of mania, both of which occurred immediately after weaning, though her hormonal levels do not appear to have been checked. On the other hand, Dr Dalton says that sometimes established depression can lift when breastfeeding stops.

National Childbirth Trust breastfeeding counsellors and mothers have been aware for some time that many mothers become depressed at the time they stop breastfeeding their child. Breastfeeding counsellor Heather Thorn noticed that in the NCT booklet on PND a number of mothers specifically mentioned that breastfeeding problems or weaning immediately preceded their depression. She says in *New Generation*, 'These comments reflect more than a minor coincidence. I realised that I had felt depressed after weaning my first child at nine months, and by talking to other mothers discovered that this can be a common reaction. Surely there is a hormonal link here.'

A few adoptive mothers suffer from PND, and this has been taken to indicate social and psychological causes for their depression, and as evidence that PND is not hormonally linked. But the opposite could be true. There have been cases of adoptive mothers who, with sufficient nipple stimulation, have been able to produce enough milk to feed the babies they did not give birth to. And the cries, smell and feel of a baby, especially with skin-to-skin contact, trigger hormonal responses in biological mothers – manifested as the let-down reflex, a surge of milk. So, even when breastfeeding is not taking place, it is possible that hearing and handling an adopted baby affects hormonal output, with prolactin being made and the hormonal balance changed, producing depressive symptoms.

Psychiatrist John Cox and Elizabeth Alder did a study in Edinburgh which considered whether breastfeeding women are more likely to suffer from PND than bottlefeeding mothers and found the pattern of breastfeeding to be an important influence. Total breastfeeders (up to 12 weeks) were found to be twice as likely to develop PND as others. Nearly half of the totally breastfeeding women had depressive symptoms and some were severely depressed. Unfortunately, 50 out of the 89 women in this study took the pill, making it difficult to disentangle the results, but none of the partially breastfeeding mothers had symptoms of depression.

However, partial breastfeeding invariably has an adverse effect on its continuation as there is insufficient stimulation to keep up milk levels, and breastfeeding has many advantages (see Chapter 7). As women already receive much conflicting advice about breastfeeding, and this is disturbing and detrimental to their efforts to continue feeding, this is an area that should be properly investigated. In the meantime, Heather Thorn advises cutting out feeds slowly, so that weaning is as leisurely as possible, to prevent sudden hormonal changes.

The contraceptive pill

This is not the place to deal with the arguments of many authorities that taking today's low dose pills involves a tiny but worthwhile risk to health (or even contain some protective factors), and others that taking the pill, at any stage of a woman's life, is a recipe for biochemical problems. Further reading on the pros and cons is recommended (see Getting Help).

When the pill had become extremely popular, Sir Charles Dodd, the British scientist who synthesised orally effective oestrogen in 1938, commented glumly, 'When a clock is working, you don't tinker with it.' In the 1970s a New York State Cancer Control Bureau doctor told the US Senate that natural or synthetic forms of oestrogen and progesterone are 'potent modifiers of biological function ... these drugs produce simultaneous effects in many systems of the body.'

In her recent book *The Bitter Pill* Dr Ellen Grant says that in early animal studies it was discovered that 'the actions of several brain hormones were blocked.' The original high dose pills produced loss of interest in lovemaking, huge swings in mood, and depression. Dr Grant says of the trials in which she was involved, 'what was obvious was that some women were much more susceptible to certain side-effects than others.'

To consider other links between the pill and PND, the artificial progestogen in the pill lowers a woman's level of her own progesterone. Taken soon after the birth of a baby, the pill perpetuates low progesterone levels – the reverse of what seems to be needed to lower the chances of PND. Mothers taking the pill are more likely to be depressed up to 3–5 months postnatally than those not on the pill (Alder and Cox). They found no differences between progestogen only (minipill) and combined pill users.

When the pill is taken postnatally, depression that occurs then may actually be a direct side-effect of the hormones in it rather than being PND. Dr Dalton considers that taking the pill may 'enhance or precipitate a state of depression'. For breastfeeding mothers, other aspects of being on the pill to consider are that the quantity and quality of their milk is likely to decrease, the duration of lactation may be shortened, and the hormones will pass through the milk to their babies. Though it is not known exactly what effects powerful synthetic hormones can have on newborns, even in tiny quantities, it seems unnecessary to take any risk.

Sensitivity to hormones

That some women are sensitive to individual sex hormones or resistant to them has been known since 1942. While levels may be normal, some part of their system reacts strongly against one hormone or does not respond when it should. Either way, the symptoms would be of a conventional hormonal problem. In 1953 Heckel's work led him to conclude that endocrine allergy is 'common rather than unusual'. And in 1974 'startling, rapid and unusually effective relief of progesterone related symptoms' was obtained by Miller, using injections of extremely small doses of progesterone. The effectiveness of the treatment was reduced or nullified when increased doses were tried.

The PMS Clinic in Dallas, Texas, find that the majority of their patients have normal, well-balanced hormone levels and says, 'it became clear that many PMS patients were simply over-sensitive to their own hormones.' The clinic also say, 'Any shock to the immune system, including infection, pregnancy or chemical exposure, can upset immune control mechanisms, allowing the inappropriate development of antibodies against things that are not normally "enemies" of the body (food, hormones, etc).'

A history of pill-taking may be another thing triggering abnormal reactions to normal endocrine levels. So may an intake from babyhood of natural oestrogens in some foods, and sex hormones fed to farm animals and poultry to make them put on weight, although this practice is being stopped within the EEC. Whatever the cause, these hidden factors complicate hormonal assessment and treatment. But if their existence is recognised and tested for, it may be found that desensitisation treatment ends hormonally linked mental disturbances, with the possibility that it can be used to treat or prevent PND.

Thyroid and adrenal involvement

While Dr Dalton's main concern has been with the pituitary/ hypothalamus endocrine system, she does say that, 'The adult with too low a hormonal output from the thyroid gland may be referred to a psychiatrist because of depression, apathy, slowness of thought, inability to concentrate, and confusion. The mind is sick, but the cause is hormonal.'

Isolated workers have suspected for a long time that PND could involve one or more of the endocrine systems of the pituitary, the thyroid and the adrenals. Following on cases which Dr Hamilton found responded well to doses of thyroxine (one of the thyroid hormones), and cases which Dr Ione Railton (also working in San Francisco) found improved with doses of prednisolone, (a substance related to the adrenal hormone cortisone), some doctors now think there is a simple sequence of hormonal events which explains the symptoms for all forms of PND.

Dr Hamilton says, 'During pregnancy many hormonal systems work at high intensity. The pituitary, very active, sends extra chemical messengers to the adrenals and thyroid and these glands work overtime. The pituitary is driven, at least partly, by the large amounts of oestrogen and progesterone, produced mainly by the placenta. At delivery the measurable levels of these hormones drop rapidly towards near-zero in 24 hours. But nothing happens, psychologically, for at least three days, usually longer. So it would appear that the illness which appears later is not a *direct* effect of the drop in oestrogen and progesterone.

'With the drop in oestrogen and progesterone, the pituitary quickly becomes sluggish, and all of its hormones decrease. In turn, the thyroid and adrenals diminish their activity, but the process is slower. In three to seven days after birth the adrenals slow down. There is a lot of the adrenal hormone cortisol remaining in the blood, but most of it is bound to a large sticky protein molecule. Only the newly-formed unbound, or free cortisol is physiologically effective. When production slows, in some women this free cortisol may

114

approach zero, with the production of psychological symptoms – early puerperal psychoses, and, maybe, in lesser degree, the blues.

'Low thyroid levels are known to produce depression, but it takes longer for thyroid to settle to a symptom-producing deficit level postnatally than it does for adrenal. Beyond the early agitation of the cortisol-deficit cases and the later depression of the thyroid-deficit cases, there are many cases which seem to combine both sets of symptoms and, in this view, the sluggish pituitary is indirectly responsible for both. The same hypotheses of early cortisol lack and later thyroid deficit apply to lesser degrees of postpartum distress, the blues early in the puerperium, and postnatal depression later.'

Unfortunately, because of the enormous expense that would be involved together with the questionable ethics of letting some women go untreated, scientific trials on thyroid and adrenal hormonal involvement in PND have not gone ahead. Dr Hamilton personally believes that 'In the interests of patients, and in getting into definitive treatment before the year 2050, we should try a variety of indirect measures to test these hypotheses. We have become paralysed by "proof" requirements which are feasible and inexpensive in the study of rat learning, but which are overly-rigid when we are trying to treat very sick women.'

Why do hormones create problems?

Hormonal levels undoubtedly affect brain chemistry and therefore mood and behaviour. But we are back to the cause and effect conundrum. We are programmed to survive, therefore to take care of our newborns and protect them from danger. We cannot do this properly if we are lethargic, distraught or downright deranged. So our bodies are meant to be able to cope while progesterone is low after birth, then go on to swiftly restore the oestrogen progesterone balance to pre-pregnancy levels, dealing fairly smoothly with the transition. If the transition is irregular or delayed in a significant number of women, this is peculiar.

I do not believe that women become anxious, depressed and disturbed because their bodies simply cannot get through the immediate postnatal period of low progesterone, with associated low levels of other hormones, or because their hormonal levels fail of their own accord to return swiftly and smoothly to pre-pregnancy levels. But rather that the 'programmed' return is actively prevented by a variety of mediating factors which may be physical or emotional. When the functioning of the various interlinked endocrine systems is hampered, a variety of mental symptoms result.

WHAT AFFECTS HORMONAL LEVELS

The mediating factors that can create problems include:

- an ill-timed, interrupted or condensed birth sequence eg amniotomy and/or hormonal induction and acceleration; timed, hurried second stage; hormones given to speed up third stage, early cutting of cord
- drugs given to kill pain
- stress during the birth – caused either by interventions, staff attitudes and hospital atmosphere, or because of problems with birth partner
- difficulties in establishing breastfeeding
- stress after the birth – because of poor housing, money problems; problems with partner; difficulty in adjusting to new life or feeling close to the baby, caused by unrealistic expectations or psychological problems, perhaps originating in childhood
- not being in close physical contact with the baby most of the time for, say, the first eight weeks
- plain, unadulterated, straightforward exhaustion, due to shortage of sleep or, worse, broken sleep pattern; large amount of household and babycare tasks
- lack of exercise, especially outdoors
- being very much overweight (as opposed to having healthy reserves)
- being underweight or attempting to diet
- being inadequately nourished, especially if breastfeeding
- food sensitivities
- environmental pollution – chemicals in food, water, air
- being on the pill
- using cigarettes, alcohol, social drugs
- taking tranquillisers or antidepressants; having ECT

EARLIER PROBLEMS

Certain other factors may indicate that hormonal functioning was less than optimal before the birth, making achieving a balance postnatally more difficult. These include:

- history of PMS
- history of pill-taking
- history of subfertility or miscarriage
- being older
- certain complications of pregnancy, particularly pre-eclampsia
- depression during pregnancy
- premature delivery and/or low birthweight infant
- previous mental illness

It seems then, that various hormonal problems are involved in causing the blues, postnatal depression and puerperal psychosis. However, hormonal problems do not happen in isolation and there are several ways of decreasing their incidence. Reducing stress of all kinds is a key aim. But there are also biochemical ways of preventing or treating hormonal imbalances which may in many instances be cheaper, easier to administer, more subtle, more appropriate and more effective than giving doses of hormones or hormone substitutes.

This approach of helping the body to correct its imbalances also has the advantage over progesterone that it can be used once depression is established. Progesterone is useful only in preventing depression, unless it is given within the first day or two of its onset. It is rare for a mother, people close to her, or medical professionals attending her to realise so quickly that something is wrong, and then these people may not be aware of or believe in progesterone therapy, so the opportunity for its use is likely to be missed.

So, what are the other biochemical methods of maintaining or restoring a favourable hormonal balance?

NUTRITION

The easiest way to help the body to function normally is to eat well. Endless arguments exist about what correct nutrition is, partly because of differences in definition. Malnourishment can mean anything from starvation to low levels of certain obscure micronutrients. Here I am talking about optimal nutrition. This is concerned with quality rather than quantity and recognises that requirements will vary from one person to the next, and according to what is happening in their life. Optimal nutrition is concerned with total intake and balance of the major nutrients – proteins, carbohydrates, fats; micronutrients – vitamins, minerals and some other key substances in food and supplements; and the sensitivities to foods and added chemicals that many people show.

There is at least general agreement that the recent British National Advisory Committee on Nutritional Education (NACNE) Report provides sensible recommendations for a varied basic diet. They advised:

- reducing fat, both the total amount and the ratio of saturated (animal) fats to polyunsaturated (vegetable) oils
- reducing sugar by half
- reducing alcohol
- reducing salt
- reducing protein from animal sources
- increasing whole grains, fruits and vegetables

Large sectors of the general public are currently showing a keen interest in what they eat, and as there is a vast amount of published information available this book does not go into more detail. Since 'health foods' are now big business, that name is given to many foods that do not deserve it, so when attempting to follow a healthy eating programme it is very important to read labels and ask questions.

One barrier to achieving optimal nutrition is lack of knowledge. Another is simply lack of money. Even when food values are understood, poverty plus lack of time and energy mean that many families do not eat the food they know would be good for them. And within the family it is invariably the wife or mother who does without so that the man and the children may have more or better quality food. During pregnancy all nutritional needs are increased, but an adequate let alone optimal diet is not possible for many women. The Maternity

Alliance calculates that the average weekly cost of an adequate diet for pregnant women represents some 32% of the supplementary benefit for a couple and 52% of that for a single woman. By the time their babies are born, many women's reserves of vitamins and minerals are depleted.

To all those who have long struggled for nutrition to take its rightful place – as a key way of ensuring physical and mental health – the tremendous early resistance among doctors to the moderate ideas in the NACNE report came as no suprise. In Britain and the USA doctors and medical staff are almost totally untrained in nutrition. It has been suggested many times that farmers, livestock specialists and veterinary surgeons are nutritionally better informed than physicians, and certainly the greatest care is taken with the diet of breeding stock – before conception, during pregnancy and throughout lactation. This contrasts with human medicine where, for example, preconceptual care has only recently been promoted. Obstetrician Dr Tom Brewer says that 'A lot of Americans feed their lawns better than their pregnant women.'

Even in fields like endocrinology where, for example in Germany, it is accepted that there is interaction between the hormonal and nervous systems and dietary factors, prominent American nutritionist Carlton Fredericks says 'such a viewpoint is largely alien to American medical thinking, which tends to view the glands as if in a vacuum.' In considering individual susceptibility to disorders he also says, 'Once diet is considered, it becomes possible to unify what otherwise appears to be an array of totally independent factors which elevate or lower resistance.' In a paper on trace elements and behaviour the American authors say, 'Trace elements have been largely ignored by all biological and behavioural scientists.'

Psychodietetics is based on the idea that a host of emotional problems, labelled as 'mental', are actually rooted in improper diet. The authors of an American book on the subject, including Dr Cheraskin, say, 'Based on mounting evidence that sound bio-chemical principles underly the food-to-mood phenomenon, and that dietary nutrients have a profound influence on the way we feel, think, respond to, and perceive the world around us, the authors conclude that nutritional therapy should be used as an adjunct to other forms of mental therapy. In many of the causes we've treated, diet alone "did the trick".'

119

Why supplements?

Maintaining an adequate, balanced intake of high quality foods is the ideal way to avoid deficiencies. However, supplements are invaluable in building up someone who has had poor nutrition, when extra stress means it is unlikely that sufficient of certain nutrients can be obtained from food, and for certain individuals who have inherited metabolic defects.

About women's particular needs, noted biochemist Dr Len Mervyn says, 'The strain of a hectic lifestyle, pressure of home versus career, the increased evidence of smoking and drinking in women, and the greater reliance on analgesics and antibiotics, all take their toll on nutritional status, by increasing the individual's requirement to way above normal levels.'

It is difficult nowadays to get adequate nutrition for ordinary needs, let alone special ones like pregnancy, birth and lactation, from the frequently recommended 'good mixed diet'. Modern farming, agricultural and food processing methods mean that much food that appears wholesome is of little nutritional value. In addition, harmful substances that rob the body of nutrients and create imbalances enter the food at various points in its production (see later).

Food and the brain

The idea of the brain needing good nutrition is considered relatively bizarre and usually ignored. Yet noted biochemist, Dr Roger J Williams, explains that brain cells, like all living cells, are commonly undernourished. 'To give them fuller and better balanced nutrition seems like an exceedingly promising way to prevent and treat mental disease.' And, 'The . . . most important way of improving the environment of the brain cells of the [mentally] afflicted or threatened individuals is to give them an opportunity of receiving the full nutritional chain of life – not an abbreviated or mutilated version. The brain cells ultimately get from the blood only those nutrient elements that are furnished in the food we eat.'

Hormones and food

Dr Guy Abraham has established that deficiency in any of a possible 50 vitamins, minerals and other nutrients can upset hormonal balance, and the Pre-Menstrual Tension Advisory Service believe that diet can deal with most PMS problems. It seems commonsense that optimal nutrition postnatally must give some protection against hormonal problems arising then, hopefully reducing the incidence of PND.

Blood sugar problems

Our bodies are simply not designed to cope with the amount of sugar we eat nowadays – neither the total volume, nor the high levels obtained at one meal through refined and processed foods. Blood sugar levels are critically linked to hormonal regulation. Dr Fredericks says, 'All forms of sugar raise vitamin need and depress the supply, and all forms cause disturbances of blood chemistry.' One of the main disturbances is hypoglycaemia and Dr Fredericks links low sex drive, neurotic behaviour, anxiety, suicidal depression and psychosis to this condition. One American doctor found that 77% of his hypoglycaemic patients suffered from depression. Elsewhere it has been associated with belligerence, poor concentration, crying, fatigue, irritability, excessive worrying, emotional instability, PMT and postpartum problems.

Insulin is a hormone that promotes the removal of sugar from the bloodstream and its storage in cells of the body. If blood sugar levels rise rapidly, too much insulin is released by the pancreas, causing a dramatic drop in blood sugar levels – hypoglycaemia. Despite understanding of this cycle and its effect on mood being well established women are often forbidden to eat during labour, then put on a glucose drip. This is done 'in case we need to use a general anaesthetic'. These women are likely to have very low blood sugar levels straight after birth, and hospital food will not stabilise them.

Another cause of hypoglycaemia is chronic stress. In response to stress the adrenal glands produce stress hormones (adrenaline and cortisone) which increase blood sugar levels to provide energy to cope with the stressful situation. When subject to chronic stress, however, the adrenal glands become exhausted. One stressor is

121

allergy, which does result in sudden fluctuations in blood sugar levels and so changes in mood. At low levels of progesterone, premenstrually and postnatally, the body reacts sooner to falling levels of blood sugar with the resulting production of adrenaline. One of the effects of this hormone is a feeling of impatience and irritability.

Low blood sugar leads to a craving for sugary foods. If these are eaten, the whole cycle starts off again. The answer is to eat frequent, small, high protein meals, and radically reduce refined flour and sugar intake in favour of complex carbohydrates (whole grains). Refined carbohydrates are a poor source of B vitamins. These are necessary for the body to use carbohydrates, so they are drawn from the body's reserves which are already low if the diet lacks whole-foods. Vitamin B complex and vitamin C reduce sugar craving. This type of diet, which provides the body and brain with a stable level of sufficient blood sugar, is advocated for avoiding depression, and Dr Dalton recommends frequent small meals or snacks for avoiding PMS.

Overweight or too thin?

Apart from aiming to follow a balanced food programme and obtain key nutrients in sufficient quantities, the sheer amount of food women need postnatally is often overlooked. It is true that a certain percentage of the population is overweight, but one group that often has too low an energy intake is young women. Those of 19 to 21 on average have less than 80% of the recommended energy intake. Young girls often diet to try to become as slim as the photographic models in magazines they read. Yet among women athletes and even heavy exercisers, the havoc low weight wreaks on the hormone system, signalled by abnormal menstrual cycles and periods, is well documented. Both a sudden reduction in food intake and being below a critical body weight are implicated.

Fortunately, women are no longer urged to diet in pregnancy, unless they have a particular weight-related health problem. Yet after birth women are still being told to 'get back to normal' as quickly as possible. Apart from this being an added, unnecessary pressure, it is usually bad advice. New mothers need a lot of energy, and a lot of high-quality food, even when they are not breastfeeding. Being a bit on the chunky side (not gross) provides reserves for this time when many demands are made on the system. Becoming slim can wait until a child is one or two, or perhaps when a nightwaker starts to give you regular unbroken sleep.

Actually, people who eat 'optimally' are rarely overweight (even if they consider themselves plump) because good nutrition allows a 'natural', stable weight to be achieved by each individual. So eating well and exercising will mean that you end up with the right amount of firm flesh.

Wonder substances

Advice on supplements is prolific, frequently confusing and, by the time it reaches the general public, often seems little more than a matter of fashionable whim, with one cure-all succeeding another in the headlines. There is no easy answer and choosing a regime of supplements without first consulting a doctor, nutritionist or qualified alternative practitioner means embarking on a course of self-education. This is perfectly possible by following the guide-lines in any number of nutritional self-help books currently available.

Problems usually occur when DIY health devotees confuse short-term very high therapeutic dosages with low level maintenance doses, or cause an imbalance between nutrients. Greatly heightened needs for micronutrients may occur that derive from the body's efforts to mobilise its resources when under stress. For example, strong emotional stress can cause the body to utilise vitamin C by the thousands of milligrams.

While there is no one tablet which, taken in isolation and in quantity, will magic away all symptoms, there are certain micro-nutrients and traditionally used plants that do have a beneficial effect on a wide variety of conditions. Vitamin C improves health generally, is frequently short in the diet, is water soluble so does not build up in the body, and most people would benefit from an intake of 1000mg a day. A warning sign that too much is being taken is persistent diahorrea.

Taking the B complex vitamins together is another general answer to feeling run down. Again, they are water soluble and most cheaper brands contain a sufficiently high dosage. Vitamin E has many devo-tees but, as it is fat soluble, levels can build up in tissues and regular doses should not exceed 100mg daily. Selenium is an essential trace mineral and is in short supply in the soil of most areas in Europe, the USA, Australia and New Zealand. A daily intake of 50mg is effective; excessive intake is dangerous.

Supplements and depression

General good health and resistance to stress is, of course, the aim of most supplementation. But it is possible to use certain nutrients and other naturally occurring substances to treat specific illnesses. Throughout history biochemical methods of alleviating the symptoms of depression have been tried, derived from various plant, animal or mineral sources. But it is only with recent advances in molecular biology, knowledge of brain chemistry and of metabolic pathways in the body that the way in which these early remedies worked and, more importantly, the chemical causes of depression are being established.

The brain is composed of millions of nerve cells or neurons. In order for the brain to control the processes of the body and mind, electrical impulses pass from one cell to another, following a pathway. There are gaps between some of the neurons along these pathways and, in order for an electrical impulse to cross the gaps it uses chemicals called neurotransmitters.

Granules of neurotransmitters are made and stored in the ends of neurons, released into the surrounding fluid when an electrical impulse reaches that point, attracted to the beginnings of the next neuron, and there broken down by the enzyme monoamine-oxidase. The neurotransmitters about which most is understood are amines called serotonin (5-HT) and noradrenaline and dopamine (both catecholamines). They all regulate behaviour, thoughts and feelings. Low levels and imbalances of these substances can cause irritability, aggression, loss of concentration, insomnia and depression of varying severity.

Supplements and PMS

Problems with neurotransmitters may be the result of an inherent biochemical defect, low levels of certain foods and micronutrients in the diet, temporary adaptations of the body's chemistry to outside factors such as stress, or endocrine changes related to the menstrual cycle or birth and lactation. For example, serotonin produces feelings of well-being. Just before a period, because of hormonal changes, levels of serotonin drop, and the symptoms of PMT can occur. A parallel low level of progesterone, affecting serotonin levels, occurs after birth.

Because of the parallels between PMS and PND, there has been much speculation as to whether certain substances that alleviate or get rid of PMS symptoms could usefully be given to PND sufferers. Dr Dalton uses progesterone, but various nutrients that are or should be present in our diet affect hormones. Researchers usually consider these in isolation, but their effectiveness is increased in combination – either with each other, or additional micronutrients.

WONDER SUBSTANCES AND PND

Naturally occurring substances recommended to alleviate mental illness, anxiety, depression or PMS/PMT act at a variety of points along metabolic pathways. The chief naturally occurring substances that have been proved to have beneficial effects on PND in some women, or on which research is currently being done, are as follows. They can all be bought without a prescription from chemists or healthfood shops or by mail order (see Getting Help).

Vitamin B6

Some of the signs of low intake or malabsorption of this vitamin are irritability, nervousness and depression. Vitamin B6 has been used to treat psychoses and, for over 10 years, to treat depression caused by taking the pill and depression in PMS. Just before a period, as a result of high oestrogen levels, serotonin levels drop and B6 helps to raise them again.

B6 is a key vitamin, involved in many metabolic pathways and needed to enable other vitamins to work. The recommended daily allowance of 2mg is low because it does not take into account substantial inborn differences in our ability to utilise B6, or increased needs when dealing with specific circumstances such as stress.

According to Dr Williams, in a sample of 800 psychiatric patients needs were said to vary from 5–400mg daily. Scientific writer Barbara Seaman and psychiatrist Gideon Seaman believe that 30–50mg a day are needed to deal with pill-induced depression, or up to 100mg when there is hypoglycaemia (see later).

Dr Michael Brush of St Thomas's Hospital, London, and the charity Women's Health Concern have been most active in researching and presenting B6 (pyridoxine) as an answer for PMS, although they stress that no one treatment will help every PMS sufferer. They recommend doses from 20–200mg a day, but 50–100mg is the most usual amount taken.

Dr Riley has studied the effects of B6 on PND. She based her work on links between PMS and PND, and PMS and B6, and the fact that B6 deficiency is common in late pregnancy (there is an increased requirement for B6 in pregnancy). She set out to test the theory that 'pyridoxine might have a short-term effect in reducing the severity of the blues, and hence a more long-term effect in the prevention of more severe and prolonged postnatal depression.' The dosage given was 100mg B6 daily for 28 days after birth. She found that 'the proportion with severe depressive symptomatology in those on active medication [B6] was only a quarter of that in patients on placebo.'

Mothers were assessed after delivery, at day 5, day 28 and one year after the birth. The group with no history of PMS became progressively less depressed at each assessment, and there was no significant difference in mean depression score between those given B6 and those given placebo tablets. In contrast, the PMS group were more depressed by day 5, though this increase was smaller in the B6 group.

'By one month the treated PMS group had a significantly lower mean depression score and, without further treatment, this improvement was maintained until the end of the first year after delivery.' Of those in the PMS group 'on active medication, 5% were cases of depression at one month and 10% at one year, whilst in the placebo PMS group there were 20% and 33% respectively.'

She concludes that PMS is predicative of vulnerability to PND, and that PND can be reduced by taking vitamin B6. She believes that if B6 were given towards the end of pregnancy, PND might be avoided or reduced in severity and is doing research on this now.

Psychiatrist Dr Carl Pfeiffer of the Brain Bio Center, New

Jersey, believes that the requirement for supplements and their levels should be 'determined by individual need'. With B6 he applies a simple test for this. Deficiency causes problems in remembering dreams; too much (or a dose taken at night) will produce 'restlessly vivid dreams and insomnia'. He personally finds 50mg a day sufficient, but can drop this to 25mg when he is on holiday and less stressed.

By taking B6 while maintaining good levels of all other vitamins in the B complex, vitamin C, zinc, magnesium and, for some people gamma-linolenic acid (see later), it is possible to maximise the take-up of B6 and minimise its dose. Magnesium is particularly important in metabolising pyridoxine. If it is in short supply, higher and higher doses of B6 are needed to achieve the same effect.

Doses of 200–600mg a day over long periods have been associated with a variety of reversible neuropathic symptoms such as numbness and tingling in the extremities of the limbs. Dr Dalton has found adverse effects in women taking 50mg a day for three months, and some cases where treatment with B6 has resulted in sensitivity to the vitamin so that subsequent small doses cause a return of symptoms. It is sensible to limit the dosage and length of use, plus be alert to the possibility of side-effects. B6 should never be taken by anyone with Parkinson's disease who is taking the drug levodopa.

Zinc

This mineral is a key micronutrient. Without it many metabolic processes cannot take place. For example, zinc is essential for the correct functioning of over 200 enzymes (proteins that speed up chemical reactions, enabling food to be utilised by the body). Shortages produce physical and mental effects. According to Dr Mervyn deficiency symptoms include: 'loss of appetite, loss of smell, mental apathy, fatigue, lazy reactions, depression after birth and lack of maternal instincts.'

Zinc is not easily mobilised from reserves in body tissues so daily intake is of great importance. The American recommended daily allowance of zinc is 15mg, of which most people get only half. It increases to 20mg for pregnant women and 25mg for nursing mothers, yet no routine supplements of zinc are given in these cases. Indeed, large doses of iron, known to hinder the absorption of zinc in the intestine, are handed out instead. Interestingly, two indications of zinc deficiency are stretch marks and nausea in pregnancy.

Zinc intake is low generally for a variety of reasons. Soils may be exhausted from overcropping and unbalanced use of fertilisers, or naturally deficient in glaciated areas (parts of northern Europe, Canada and America and South Island, New Zealand). Some food processing removes zinc. Vegetarians or those with diets low in animal protein are liable to have low zinc levels.

Toxic metals absorbed from food and the environment, particularly cadmium, mercury and lead, interfere with zinc's work in the body. When zinc levels are low to start with, these metals can accumulate to levels that produce mental disturbances, sometimes very severe. Levels of minerals and toxic metals in the body can be checked by laboratory analysis (see Getting Help).

When, for a variety of reasons, copper levels increase in blood plasma this makes the low zinc situation worse. The uptake of zinc by the plasma proteins from the intestinal walls is impaired, so the body cannot absorb what zinc is present in food. However, copper levels can be reduced by raising zinc intake above a critical level. The zinc is then able to increase copper excretion; taking manganese and vitamin B6 with zinc will speed up the process.

High ratios of copper to zinc can be caused by low zinc or high copper intake. Copper levels may be raised in contraceptive pill takers and women fitted with copper IUDs. In acid (soft) water areas tap water that has been through copper pipes is another source of copper, and the metal is added in the processing and storage of foods, and used in pesticides and fungicides, of which there are residues in foods.

Links have been established between zinc/copper levels and mental states generally. For example, high serum copper levels have been found in manic depressives. When kidney patients on dialysis machines accidentally accumulate excess copper in the blood, they develop temporary psychiatric symptoms of unreality, disperceptions and even psychosis. At the time in their cycle that women suffer from PMS, which often includes depression and outbursts of aggression, zinc levels are low while copper levels are high. According to Dr Pfeiffer the stress of an operation frequently depletes the body's stores of zinc. Post-operative depression is common and it is worth noting that rates of PND are higher after caesarean births.

Pregnancy and birth have a marked effect on zinc/copper levels, causing a change in ratios or making an existing imbalance worse. Dr Ellen Grant points out, 'A pregnant and lactating woman needs extra zinc for her growing child. Zinc is concentrated in the placenta and lost at childbirth.' There is 360–600mg of zinc in a healthy fullterm placenta and this loss needs to be made up fast. Animal mothers eat their placentas and within some 96 hours of giving birth their zinc/copper balance is restored, and their milk contains adequate zinc to supply their offsprings' needs. Placental replacement zinc supplementation could be necessary for humans.

On the role of the pill Dr Grant says, 'If a woman has been taking the pill she is more likely to be deficient at the start of her pregnancy. As zinc supplements are not usually taken by most pregnant mothers, this means that postpartum zinc deficiency, severe enough to induce depression, will have become more common among mothers.'

Dr Pfeiffer has found many depressed patients high in serum copper. He also postulates a link between high copper (implying low zinc) and PND. Copper levels are elevated by oestrogen, the output of which increases greatly in pregnancy. Serum copper is more than twice as high at delivery as at conception and this takes two or three months to drop back down again. He says, 'This high postpartum copper level may be a factor in causing postpartum depression and psychosis; more data are needed in this area.'

Low zinc levels (before, during and after pregnancy), allergy and depression are also linked. As zinc is necessary for enzyme systems to metabolise particular foods, when insufficient zinc is available and they are not fully broken down, allergic reactions to these foods can occur that cause mental disturbances in some people (see later). Conversely, allergic reactions to foods, 'alien' proteins and chemicals cause an increase in certain white blood cells called eosinophils. They contain 250 times more zinc than other white blood cells, so allergic reactions 'mop up' a lot of zinc, making less available for other needs.

Derek Bryce-Smith, professor of organic chemistry at Reading University, together with medical colleagues has been involved in both research and clinical work using zinc. A simple taste test is used: those who cannot taste a weak solution of zinc are usually deficient. Professor Bryce-Smith says, '[We] find that the majority of depressives are unable to taste the solution, and show a beneficial response to supplementation.'

He goes on to say, 'Stress in general causes increased loss of zinc ... it seems reasonable to suppose that the trauma of birth plus the loss of zinc in the placenta could in some cases precipitate a state of clinical zinc deficiency. Mental depression is well known to be one of the symptoms of such a condition ... I do not suggest that all cases of postnatal depression result from zinc deficiency, but I am satisfied that a significant proportion of cases are either caused or exacerbated by this'. He therefore suggests that the taste test should be given in all cases of PND, and has devised a combination test kit and zinc supplement that can be bought by the general public (see Getting Help).

Because zinc deficiency kills taste, a yearning for strong-tasting foods and the habit of salting everything heavily in an attempt to add taste is a good rule-of-thumb indicator that zinc levels could be low.

Evening primrose oil

One possible cause of hormonal imbalance or abnormal levels persisting after birth is a shortage in the diet of a particular fatty acid called gamma-linolenic acid (GLA). GLA seems to be another 'wonder substance' that will relieve or stop a very wide range of symptoms, physical and mental, when given in supplement form, usually as oil from the evening primrose plant.

The way in which GLA acts, and the reasons why deficiencies are widespread, are complicated. GLA is derived from essential fatty acids (EFAs), commonly called polyunsaturates. We have been warned for years that our diets are too high in saturated animal fats and too low in polyunsaturated plant oils, and many people have corrected this balance. They get enough of the most important EFA, linoleic acid, so should not be GLA deficient. But linoleic acid is useless unless it is present in cis-linoleic form and other factors allow it to be converted to GLA.

A lot of things can prevent this. They include:

- too much saturated animal fat
- conversion of cis-linoleic acid, by heating, hydrogenating or other processing, to trans-linoleic acid
- alcohol consumption
- food additives
- high levels of the hormone adrenaline, made in response to stress
- low levels of zinc, magnesium and vitamin B6

GLA is so vital because it is further converted, first to dihomo-gamma-linolenic acid (DGLA) then to prostaglandin E1 (PGE1). Prostaglandins are a powerful group of substances, occurring in most tissues, that mimic hormonal activity and so have a variety of complex actions. PGE1 has a list of effects, two of which are producing a sense of well-being and relieving the symptoms of PMS. As there are many problems in getting sufficient levels of GLA in the diet one short cut to obtaining its benefits is to take evening primrose oil (EPO) supplements.

Patients with depression have been found to produce less PGE1 than normal. Dr David Horrobin says, 'The brain is exceptionally rich in precursor essential fatty acids from which prostaglandins are derived and PGs are known to be produced by brain tissue and to regulate nerve conduction, transmitter release and transmitter acceptance. Their basic biochemistry and physiology makes PGs candidates for regulators of behaviour in the way that the catecholamines or other neurotransmitters are.'

The most popularly known effects of EPO are on PMS. Too little GLA, and so PGE1, can make a woman's body hypersensitive to changes in hormonal levels, causing PMS symptoms. EPO raises GLA and therefore PGE1 levels. The best effects are produced when a number of co-factors are taken at the same time. These are vitamin B6, niacin (B3), vitamin C, zinc and magnesium, plus vitamin E and selenium.

Dr Michael Brush found in trials that EPO produced relief in all but 15% of women who had failed to respond to other treatments. Two 500mg Efamol capsules were given twice daily after food, continuously in the worst cases, but three days before the expected start of symptoms in most. The treatment has now been taken up by many clinics and individual doctors, through it is still unknown to or ignored by many.

As EPO relieves PMS symptoms and can produce 'a modest euphoria', there has been much speculation as to whether it could be used to treat or avoid PND. Many women who have found EPO helpful with PMS, or read about it, have then either tried it when they had PND or recommended it to other depressed mothers. Word of mouth reports, especially among NCT mothers, are that results are encouragingly good. Because of this interest, and because of the known links between PMS and PND, one manufacturer of EPO supplements, Efamol are currently engaged in trials. Dr Horrobin is their clinical research director and says these trials are 'looking at the effects of Efamol in the postnatal period, with depression being one of the things which is being monitored.'

The oily nature of EPO can cause slight indigestion, and some people react to other substances in the capsules. It is variously available as 250mg or 500mg capsules, in 10ml dropper bottles, or in tablet form (see Getting Help) which may offer better absorption of GLA. EPO sometimes causes headaches. This could happen when an individual is zinc deficient and EPO is best taken with its co-nutrients. Anyone with epilepsy should not take EPO.

Amino acids

These organic compounds form the chief constituents of protein. They can be split off from the chain of molecules of protein and, in this free form, are used as nutritional supplements, among other things to treat food sensitivities. But their greatest potential use seems to be in the effect they have on mental and emotional states. American psychologist and nutritional expert Dr Robert Erdmann believes that 'carefully selected free amino acids will prove to be the psychiatric treatment of the future.'

Amino acids, whether absorbed from animal or vegetable foods or from supplements, supply the raw materials for making hormones and neurotransmitters. *Harpers & Queen* health editor Leslie Kenton says, 'Amino acid therapy is based on the hypothesis that if the dynamic pool of nutrients needed for healthy brain functioning is complete, then mental and emotional aberrations will be rare. It treats psychiatric symptoms by analysing the patient's biochemical imbalances and then restoring them by way of sophisticated nutritional programmes.' Carefully selected amino acids are taken with their vitamin and mineral co-factors. Because free-form amino acid supplements require no digestion, they are absorbed into the bloodstream immediately and produce an effect in days or even hours.

Tryptophan is present in protein foods such as milk, fish and soya beans and available as a health food supplement in tablet form. L-tryptophan enters the brain where it is converted into the neurotransmitter serotonin. Given as a supplement, this amino acid has been used to treat sleeplessness, anxiety and depression, the last with varying degrees of success. Results improve when L-tryptophan

132

is given with vitamins B1, B2, B6 and niacin (B3). These have an antidepressant effect of their own, and niacin allows the effective tryptophan dose to be reduced by one third. A daily dose of 1g, taken after the evening meal, has been found to relieve depression, but it has been used in clinical trials in doses as high as 3g a day. Excessive intake can result in feeling muzzy-headed and drowsy. L-tryptophan should not be taken during pregnancy.

Tyrosine can be used as a supplement to produce neurotransmitters that stimulate mental activity. However, a breakdown product of tyrosine, tyramine, can create problems. Tyramine is present in cheese, wine, yeast extract and a list of other foods and can result in severe migraine-type headaches in sensitive individuals. The enzyme monoamine oxidase destroys tyramine before it reaches the bloodstream. If MAO inhibiting antidepressants (see Chapter 5) are taken, tyramine circulates in the bloodstream, raising blood pressure to cause blinding headaches and sometimes fatal brain haemorrhage.

A team at the Institute of Obstetrics and Gynaecology, based at Queen Charlotte's Maternity Hospital, London, and headed by Professor Merton Sandler, have been working on links between depression and tyramine (although their research began as an examination of migraines). As well as being destroyed by MAO, tyramine can be deactivated by other processes in the body. Professor Sandler has found that people with an unusually low ability to deactivate tyramine are vulnerable to endogenous depression (where biochemical changes can be more clearly demonstrated than with so-called neurotic depression).

Professor Sandler originally thought that a test the team devised, which shows how much tyramine an individual can metabolise before it reaches the bloodstream, could be used to predict which pregnant women are likely to suffer from PND. He now feels it cannot be used in this way as he considers he has confirmed PND should be categorised as neurotic, not endogenous.

DLPA is an amino acid which is thought to have three separate antidepressant effects. First, it can be converted to a neurotransmitter-type substance which bears a close resemblance to the stimulant drug amphetamine. Second, DLPA can inhibit enzymes which break down endorphins. These are morphine-like hormones which can produce euphoria (see Chapter 2). Clinical research has shown that endorphins administered intravenously can trigger sudden, dramatic antidepressant actions, even in suicidal patients. The action of DLPA enables endorphins to exert their effects for longer. Third, DPLA may be converted to the brain neurotransmitter norepinephrine, a deficiency of which causes depression. In a double-blind controlled study DLPA was found to be equally as effective as the most commonly prescribed tricyclic antidepressant, imipramine. Reports from clinical investigations have also revealed that over 80% of all patients suffering from PMS have experienced good to complete relief.

ALLERGIES

How can allergies be linked to PND? In two ways. When the body is sensitive to certain substances the resulting biochemical reactions can include alterations in hormonal levels and ratios. Then pregnancy itself, stress caused by a difficult or unhappy birth, plus coping in the postnatal period can be the factors that overload a system that is already being strained, causing a previously masked sensitivity to surface, with a variety of symptoms, including depression.

The subject of allergies is another medical minefield. Learned opinions vary from 'they don't exist', to 'allergy, next to infection, is probably the most common cause of human symptomatology' (Albert Rowe, 1937) and the claim that one third of common diseases seen by GPs can be directly traced to food and chemical hypersensitivity, while these causes are partially responsible for another third of cases.

Although allergic reactions are now more often accepted as the cause of physical symptoms, it has been a long uphill struggle for those who believe that they cause mental symptoms, too. As Robert Eagle says in his book *Eating and Allergy*, 'Unfortunately the main characteristic of orthodoxy is inertia. Those with power and influence do not take kindly to having their own cherished concepts of what is what challenged.'

The ongoing and frequently bitter controversy is not helped by the confusion of terms. Many people who have symptoms that disappear when an offending food or environmental substance is removed do not exhibit the biochemical responses that conventionally show the immune system is involved. These people should properly be described as having intolerances or sensitivities, but allergy is a short, useful, evocative word and here to stay.

134

So called allergic responses fall into three broad categories:

- true allergies, causing a range of immunological responses
- a degree of poisoning because the body is dealing with toxins
- enzyme deficiency so food is not broken down properly by the digestive system

An immune response is 'the reaction to and interaction with substances interpreted by the body as not-self.' The alien substances are called antigens. In the bloodstream they meet and interact with white blood cells called B-lymphocytes which then produce antibodies. There are also white blood cells which seek out foreign proteins or invading organisms and destroy them directly.

Individuals vary enormously in what they are allergic to and the effects allergies have. Reactions can be sudden, severe and dangerous, but most are much less dramatic, producing vague symptoms, often a general feeling of being unwell and rather negative about life. Constantly responding to alien substances is a strain on the immune system which may start to give up, producing more unpleasant symptoms. Substances to which individuals are sensitive but not strictly allergic can still disturb biochemical functioning and cause a range of symptoms.

Allergy and the mind

The mental symptoms of sensitivites and allergies can range from hyperactivity and lack of concentration to amnesia, mild depression and severe mental illness. One link between allergy and mental illness is histamines. An excess of this chemical is produced when the body comes in contact with substances to which it is sensitive. Histamine, which also functions as a neurotransmitter, bypasses the blood-brain barrier and high levels can produce suicidal depression.

Dr William J Rae, a cardiovascular surgeon involved with the Dallas Environmental Control Unit, says that blood vessel damage is one early sign of environmental sensitivities. Linking this to hormonal problems he says if the early signs can be pointed out, they can be 'headed off before someone gets endocrine failure.' In noting that a reaction to beef caused one woman not only to develop spontaneous bruising but to become psychotic for two days, he speculates that vascular involvement could affect the brain, too.

New York psychiatrist Dr H L Newbold, with others, has produced work on 'ecological mental illness' or psychiatric syndromes produced by sensitivities. In testing a group of neurotics, 'common symptoms such as phobias of numerous types, hyperventilation, depression, anxiety, weakness and lethargy, hyperactivity, and numerous other common neurotic symptoms were observed as reactions to foods and commonly contacted chemicals.' This group of practitioners says, 'There is no end to the examples which the authors could give from their practice, illustrating the clinical importance of allergies producing psychiatric symptoms.'

Allergies and hormones

'Hormones are the first line of defence against allergies and become unbalanced in their efforts to fight the supposed foreign body. Women suffering from premenstrual tension, postnatal depression or menopausal symptoms may already be using their supply of hormones in counteracting hitherto undiagnosed allergies and therefore have an inadequate supply when they are needed in extra amounts at these special times,' say Mrs Ellen Rothera of the Food and Chemical Allergy Association.

The Premenstrual Syndrome Clinic in Dallas, together with the associated Environmental Control Unit, have found many connections between allergy, stress and hormones. Certain changes in hormonal levels are normal, and so are the reactions to them. When these reactions become extreme this is evidence of disorder but 'many other internal and external factors contribute to disorder in each individual. Therefore, the total load of stress on the body must be considered for effective treatment.'

Stress is any influence which upsets the body's natural smooth biochemical functioning. Stressors producing a total load include food and environmental sensitivities and demanding changes in circumstances, such as pregnancy and birth. With a build-up of stress factors the immune system is taken to its limits – a woman may even start reacting to her own hormones. 'Continued exposure causes your immune system to exceed its adaptative capacity. In this unstable condition a range of symptoms, including mental ones, is produced.'

Obviously the way to stop these problems is not to attempt to treat the specific effects, for instance with antidepressants or ECT, but to eliminate the causes. Once you read the lists of allergenic agents and start to discover what a flood of information on diet and environment exists you may feel dismayed at the scope and complexity of the problem. The advice of the Environmental Control Unit is, 'True, the problem is complex; but fortunately you have only to be concerned with simplicity itself. Your goal should be to eliminate those huge lists of chemicals from your life and to simplify your environmental stresses until you – not your environment – are in control of your health.'

The other approach of tracking down what is causing reactions in certain individuals can involve painstaking and time-consuming detective work. Fortunately, though, testing well-known allergens of all categories is simple. First avoid them completely for some three weeks. If symptoms clear, check that you have found the culprit by small re-exposure, which should promptly reactivate symptoms (sometimes unpleasantly strongly).

Candida

Candida albicans is the organism that is responsible for the vaginal infection called thrush. As well as being found in the vagina, candida is normally present in everyone's intestines as part of the flora and fauna that co-exist there and usually do not give any trouble. In certain conditions, however, it can multiply enormously and, more seriously, it can change from a simple yeast form into a mycelial fungal form. This means that it develops long root-like structures that penetrate the bowel wall, allowing incompletely digested foods, toxic candida by-products and probably the candida organism itself into the bloodstream. This can result in a wide variety of allergic-type symptoms, including emotional and mental disturbances, and candida infections have also been linked with PMS.

Antibiotics are one cause of candida overgrowth as they weaken or destroy the bacteria in the intestines that help to control it. The contraceptive pill favours its growth by altering the hormonal balance and blood sugar metabolism – yeasts thrive on sugar.

Thrush often flares up during pregnancy because of the changes in hormonal levels, particularly the very high oestrogen levels. Unchecked, candida may change to its invasive form. This change will be encouraged by sugary and refined carbohydrate foods – chosen by the pregnant woman because she craves sugar and may not realise the problems that result. Postnatally the entrenched candida will be encouraged by the same poor food – eaten from lack of choice in hospital or later from convenience because a mother is busy and fatigued. The resulting mental disturbances may be diagnosed as PND.

A bad dose of thrush may be treated with antifungal pessaries, and intestinal candida reduced by oral antifungal drugs, but the infection can be controlled by a wholefood/minimal sugar diet, plus avoiding mushrooms and foods containing yeast or other moulds (including bread, cakes, cheese, alcoholic drinks and yeast tablets). Nutritional supplements can be used to reduce the candida to a manageable level and keep it there and the bowel can be repopulated with 'friendly' bacteria in powder form.

Social poisons

We choose to use certain substances because they give us pleasure in the short-term. Sadly the pleasure is paid for, pretty quickly, with unpleasant consequences. While the proportion of users who are allergic to alcohol, tobacco and various drugs is unknown, they certainly all stress and disturb biochemical functioning and affect mental states. All these poisons also reach babies in the womb and breastfed babies and are likely to affect their behaviour. For example, Peter Fried, professor of psychology at Ottawa's Carleton University, says, 'If marijuana is used on a daily level we find stuff in the newborn. Increased tremor, exaggerated startle, altered visual response, and slightly shortened gestation are among the side-effects.' These factors make it more difficult for the mother to deal with her baby which can have links with PND (see Chapter 2).

Alcohol Cravings for this may be a result of blood sugar disturbances (see earlier), and alcohol certainly makes these worse. Indeed, some authorities consider alcoholism to be a result of errors in blood sugar metabolism, either inherited or produced by long-term poor nutrition. Alcohol uses up nutrients for its metabolism, depriving the brain cells of the benefit of those nutrients. As it is a poison, in large quantities it damages brain cells and liver cells (disturbed liver function is a cause of depression). The adverse effects of alcohol on mood and behaviour are made worse because certain drinks, particularly cheap wines, contain a wide range of chemical additives. Consumption of alcohol has risen steadily, just about doubling in the UK since 1950. Women's drinking rates have increased more sharply than men's, with the number of women diagnosed as problem drinkers having trebled in the last eight years. Women's systems are more susceptible to interference and damaging side-effects from alcohol than men's.

Cigarettes Some 40% of adults still smoke tobacco and the proportion of women who are heavy smokers did not drop between 1972 and 1982. Apart from causing over 100,000 deaths a year, and adversely affecting the health of foetuses and children, smoking causes metabolic changes that affect mood. It depletes the body of nutrients, damages the cardiovascular system (including blood vessels that supply the brain and within it), disturbs the immune system and compounds allergy problems.

Drugs The devastating effects of heroin addiction do not require elaboration. Irregular social use of cocaine and other drugs, including cannabis, usually becomes steadily more regular. All drugs upset smooth metabolic functioning, some quite dramatically. Most drugs are cut with unknown proportions of unknown substances; cannabis can be contaminated with pesticides or moulds. As with anything else, it is possible for an individual to be biochemically intolerant of a drug.

Food sensitivities

In considering allergenic factors that may be triggering or worsening PND, there are two main categories to check – foods and environmental chemicals. 'Nutrition normally affects the brain and the brain components that most markedly exhibit the effects of nutrition are neurotransmitters,' says Professor Richard J Wurtman of the Massachusetts Institute of Technology.

Milk, wheat and eggs are the foods that most commonly cause a reaction. Salicylates, in apples, blackberries, grapes, oranges, strawberries, tomatoes, for example, are another common trigger. There seems to be an increase in the number of people allergic to soya, possibly because it is so extensively used by the food industry that exposure is constantly repeated.

When trying to eliminate a food, it is important to realise that basic foods crop up again and again in hidden form in processed packaged foods, for example whey powder from milk in most bought baked goods. It is also very important to avoid all stale food as contaminating growths of moulds may be the cause of allergies, rather than the food they are growing on. Rancid fats and oils may cause reactions, too.

Mrs Gwynneth Hemmings of the Schizophrenia Association of Great Britain suffered from puerperal psychosis. She says, 'It was terrifying, but I came through with no doctor and no drugs . . . If I had known what I know now about diet I would have stuck firmly to a cereal grain free, milk-free, and probably potato and caffeine-free diet.' Her organisation feels that there should be much more research into the links between diet and mental illness.

Environmental triggers

The modern chemical industry has revolutionised our lives. We eat and are surrounded by a variety and complexity of chemicals that humankind have never been exposed to in their history. No one knows the long-term cumulative effects of most of these substances, nor what their interactions within the body can be.

Reactions to what we eat are often not caused by the food itself but by additives (preservatives, colourings, flavourings, anti-oxidants, stabilisers, thickeners, texturisers, emulsifiers), residues of agricultural chemicals, or contamination from wrapping, storage or cooking vessels.

According to the London Food Commission we now eat an average 8lb of additive chemicals a year, and this figure is growing as 75% of the average diet is made up of processed foods. The *Sunday Times* reports that a full dinner with wine can contain at least 72 additives. One loaf of our daily bread can contain a cocktail of 37 added chemicals.

Only 10% of the thousands of additives available are legally controlled. Many in use in Britain have been banned or severely restricted in America and in other parts of Europe. As Carlton Fredericks says, 'we test them individually but we swallow them together', so we do not know about their interactions. Additives are allegedly used to improve food but frequently mask a decline in

140

nutritional value and taste and are adulteration.

Britain is also notoriously lax about controlling the use of pesticides and herbicides. Friends of the Earth say, 'It is now impossible to get away from pesticides, 97–99% of all our vegetables and cereals are sprayed with one or more pesticides. Vegetables receive as many as 46 applications in a season, yet residues are hardly monitored and there are no legal limits. Up to 64% of the pesticide applied to wheat may end up unaltered in your loaf of bread.' Pesticides are neurotoxins and dissolve more easily in fats. They can reach a level of up to 300 times the blood concentration in the fats of the brain tissue.

All around us are a host of chemicals – in the air, the water, the home and at work. Apart from avoiding using any product that is not essential and, where possible, making an effort not to inhale fumes, there are certain ways of reducing the total load on the body. Drinking bottled rather than tap water where possible will help, as will using a water filter (see Getting Help). North sea gas, which has a chemical called mercaptan added to make it smell, can cause a range of mental symptoms and severe sufferers have to shut off the gas permanently.

A 19th-century battle about the use of amalgam dental fillings has resumed now that there is fresh evidence that blood levels of toxic mercury are rising and one cause is absorption from dental fillings. Preliminary data from American research suggests that 'dental amalgam and dental nickel alloys can adversely affect the quantity of T-lymphocytes.'

Jean Robinson of the Patients Association and AIMS says in *New Generation*, 'Female illnesses are often supposed to be psychosomatic, whereas men appearing with the same symptoms will be treated more "seriously". Anything that affects the hormones affects behaviour and will usually be treated as psychogenic disease and therefore the search for the toxic cause is not carried out. The study of occupational disease does not include housework and yet this is very often a missed cause of illness . . . Postnatal depression could well be classified as an occupational disease.'

Viral infections

Anyone whose immune system is weakened by reacting to allergens is likely to be more susceptible to infections, including those that are viral, and people with viral infections often find they develop allergies. One early symptom of many viral infections is a vague feeling of being down, while severe attacks can produce extreme irritability, violent mood swings and suicidal depression. In turn, 'A depressed person has depressed immune function,' says Dr Jonathan Brostoff, an immunologist at the Middlesex Hospital in London. The presence of the virulent form of candida has a role to play here, as well. As it causes or worsens allergies, the total load on the immune system is increased, making it harder for the body to throw off infections. And it is possible that candida alters the environment in the gut in a way that allows enteroviruses to take a hold there.

This group of interlinked factors is of particular relevance to new mothers. Firstly, pregnancy affects the immune system and, either because of this or because they are physically exhausted, women seem especially prone to viral infections such as glandular fever (infectious mononucleosis) in the postnatal period. Then the sort of emotional adjustments and strains that new mothers may have to work through postnatally also act as a stress on the immune system, weakening defences against allergies and infections. Viral infections, especially if they are mild, easily remain undiagnosed, in which case the mental symptoms could well be put down to PND.

Even where a viral infection was originally considered by her doctor, if the symptoms do not clear up a mother may than be suspected of mental disturbance and treated with antidepressants or pyschotherapy. It is rarely that a diagnosis of the long-lasting postviral fatigue sydrome (also known as myalgic encephalomyelitis) is thought of. The mother's many and varied but genuine physical symptoms, most noticably extreme muscular fatigue, may be brushed aside as 'all in the mind', further evidence that she has PND.

A COMPREHENSIVE APPROACH

When biochemical influences are ignored, depression and other mental changes occurring postnatally are likely to be treated by medical psychiatric intervention (drugs and ECT) or psychotherapy/ psychoanalysis – with variable results and the likelihood of recurrence over the two years following birth, after subsequent pregnancies, or throughout a lifetime. On the contrary, aiming at optimal nutrition, through diet and supplements, seems one promising way of dealing with PND. Robert Erdmann says, 'Like it or not, [humans are biochemical beings] whose biochemistry can be influenced nutritionally for better or worse. Brain changes . . . are not the simple accident of nature which many people believe.' And Dr Williams argues, 'We need to ask, What is *nature's* way of preventing mental disease? Can we, by co-operating with nature, prevent and treat mental disease successfully?'

There are five main reasons why ignoring nutrition and substances that poison the body or stress the immune system can lead to depression in the postnatal period.

High levels of toxic metals, polluting food, water and air, constantly drive down levels of essential minerals. During pregnancy large quantities of essential minerals are taken up by the baby and the placenta.

Unfavourable zinc/copper balance Zinc levels are likely to be low before pregnancy and copper levels may be rather high. During pregnancy zinc is required for the baby and 'pours itself into the placenta', while the large amount of oestrogen elevates copper levels. Zinc levels affect hormonal output while low zinc/high copper levels have been found to cause depression and mental disturbance.

Lack of B complex vitamins is a potent cause of depression and a diet of processed foods provides perhaps one quarter of our B vitamins needs. Stress resistance necessitates a high daily intake of B vitamins, and pregnant women and new mothers face a lot of pressures (see Chapter 3). After birth, while the body is rebalancing itself, there is a great need to be very peaceful. The birth, stay in hospital (see Chapter 2) and postnatal period at home are all too rarely that.

Allergies cause stress to the system and increase the requirements for key nutrients. Sensitive reactions may emerge during pregnancy.

Social poisons increase nutritional needs, which are high in pregnancy anyway.

So what measures could prevent PND? Mrs Belinda Barnes has been greatly interested in nutrition pre-pregnancy and during pregnancy for many years and founded Foresight, which promotes preconceptual care and offers nutritional guidelines for mothers after birth. As far as she knows there has been no reported incident of PND among the large numbers of mothers who have received help from Foresight preconceptually. She attributes this to Foresight's principles, as practised by their doctors (see Getting Help).

I suggest a programme I have based on the principles and methods used by Foresight. The programme should ideally be started preconceptually and continued during pregnancy and for some nine months after birth, especially if the mother is breastfeeding. Much advice is given about 'good diet' in pregnancy and when breastfeeding but it does not usually touch on most of the points explained in this chapter. And the critical time immediately following the birth is always ignored. I believe that restoring and maintaining an optimal level of nutrients from straight after birth has a key role to play in avoiding or minimising PND.

ANTI-PND DIET PROGRAMME

Toxic metals Avoid the sources of these and, if necessary, take specific supplements to lower body levels. High concentrations of toxic metals and low levels of essential minerals can be checked by blood, sweat and hair analyses.

Mineral balance Put this right through improving the basic diet and through supplementation. Pay particular attention to zinc levels.

Stress Protect against this through a wholefood diet and supplements. Many women have very packed lives and if we enrich our lives it makes sense to enrich our diets commensurately. Emotional stress is hard to avoid but it is possible to recognise and resist unnecessary pressures.

Allergies Identify allergies and decide on an appropriate course of action (avoidance, dietary supplements, desensitisation, treating candida). When mineral balance is corrected, allergies often cease to be a problem.

Social poisons Avoid alcohol, cigarettes, street drugs, unnecessary medical drugs, the contraceptive pill, copper IUDs.

Supplements As well as eating sufficient high-quality food, take specially formulated multivitamin and multimineral preparations, plus additional individual nutrients (such as evening primrose oil) where necessary. Dr Cheraskin says, 'it cannot be over-emphasised, all nutrients are interrelated . . . the optimal functioning of every single nutrient is dependent on the presence of every other essential nutrient.'

Chapter 5

Who are the carers?

The professional qualifications and chosen methods of those who end up dealing with mothers who start to behave strangely after giving birth to a baby are a matter of luck and governed by the range of local facilities plus who first decides a mother needs help. Acknowledgement that a mother feels overwhelmed or is disturbed, plus sympathy and support, are very important and mark the turning point on the road to recovery. But advice that PND is 'easily treated' may misleadingly promote false expectations – results are very variable. While most mothers can be got to function fairly well again, reasonably quickly, few would say that they felt 'normal' again for a long time after that.

What 'treatment' any mother should receive is hotly debated. But the idea that she should have treatment is never doubted. 'They consider absolutely the worst crime is doing nothing,' says one psychotherapist. The compulsion to act, to do something, no matter what, may be the psychological equivalent to 'meddlesome midwifery'. It is questionable whether any particular treatment produces improvements and cure or whether time would have done this, anyway.

As in anything else, intervention may be ineffective or actually harmful. Treading delicately and warily seems the only valid course when so little is known about the workings of the mind or brain. Talking about pharmacological cures for psychological problems in *Paper Doctors* Dr Vernon Coleman says, 'Many researchers in this field are confident that within a few years they will be able to control most human emotions with the aid of specific drugs, although they admit that they must first come to a more complete understanding of biochemical and electrical pathways within the brain . . . acquiring a total understanding of the way the brain works is likely to be a slow business. The brain contains three times as many cells as there are

145

human beings on the earth and these cells are interconnected by a series of electronic and biochemical pathways which make even the most sophisticated modern computer look like an abacus ... In addition, there are philosophical problems, for some believe that it is quite impossible for the human brain ever to completely understand itself.'

Efforts to evolve effective ways of dealing with PND are hampered by the Western 'scientific' passion for breaking everything down into its component parts and viewing these in isolation. One main division is between mind and body, with both camps fighting for ownership of the brain. As brain, body and mind have no meaning without each other, studying the ways they work together would be more useful to understanding and cure of mental disturbance than viewing them independently, as presently tends to be the case. Equally, considering illness in the individual without placing that person in the context of the world around them is a vain exercise.

One other limiting consequence of the obsession with fragmentation is that it leads to reassembling the parts in a linear model of order, with one being seen as first and most important while the others are allocated a descending order of priority. In fact, modern physics has changed the definition of the word 'scientific'. It has been necessary to abandon oversimplified models of our world and its systems, rigid separations such as that between objective and subjective, and the comfortable idea that patient study will be rewarded with the discovery of immutable laws. Instead, new dimensions, uncertainties and paradoxes have had to be embraced. Many medical practitioners, however seem to be still fighting the old battle to separate medicine from magic and to be locked into a very Victorian view of what the word scientific implies.

The seal of approval for medical (including psychiatric) treatments is usually a series of 'scientific' studies. Scientists pride themselves on their objectivity and neutrality, but objectivity is actually a philosophical impossibility. To be human and live in a given time and place is to have opinions that govern what we see. To choose a subject to study and to set up and carry out an experiment is to interfere with what is being observed. Only crude results are possible. They can act as guides or indicators but are inherently flawed and fallible.

An open mind is the only guard against blind reliance on what is considered to be proven wisdom and against perpetuating errors.

Unfortunately, becoming a professional all too often involves under-going a process of having the mind closed, through the actual training and by absorbing the values of the chosen circle. Most women who are emotionally or mentally disturbed postnatally are thought to need 'professional' help. Some support groups of 'mere' mothers go to great lengths to stress that they have 'professional' guidance. Professional may equate with being very experienced in dealing with certain problems, which can balance the limiting aspects of training, but not necessarily.

One more way in which the search for effective ways of preventing or dealing with PND is hampered and limited is that it is a woman's experience, yet everything about it is male-defined. This means that treatments are, to say the least, likely to be inappropriate. Women who are disturbed are hampered in realising that anything is wrong, then understanding what is wrong, why and what they can do about it, by living in a world that operates through male-defined language and concepts and is male-organised. Professionals who want to help these women are limited by the same constraints on analysis, communica-tion and action.

Professional help

So, who are these professionals who may or may not be able to help disturbed mothers to a greater or lesser degree? In hospital, after the birth, *the midwife* is on the alert for signs of distress. Shortlived postnatal blues will be dealt with by reassurance; severe disturbance will warrant calling in a psychiatrist. Returning home, some time in the first six weeks the mother can encounter any members of the *pri-mary health care team* – the GP, health visitor, community midwife or others (see later). If she develops depression her GP may treat her, or may refer her to a psychiatrist or other professional they consider suit-able. If a mother develops puerperal psychosis she is likely to be hospitalised where she will be under the care of a psychiatrist but meet other professionals. A few women will end up being treated by doctors who specialise in hormonal function, or nutritionists (see Chapter 4), or through various forms of complementary medicine (see Chapter 7.)

The training and functions of the various 'mind specialists' are a blur to most people, and their theories, beliefs and work do, indeed, overlap.

Psychiatrists are 'medically qualified to treat diseases of the mind' and psychiatry is 'the branch of medicine that deals with the study, treatment and prevention of mental illness'. To see a psychiatrist is therefore, to be defined as ill. GPs regularly refer their patients to a limited number of local consultant psychiatrists who work in a psychiatric hospital or psychiatric wards of a general hospital, depending on the way local services are organised. The GP may know very little about the methods any individual psychiatrist employs. Psychiatrists vary enormously in how they treat their patients – 26 'schools' of thought are listed in one medical dictionary. Some psychiatrists use physical treatments (drugs and electroconvulsive therapy), some use 'talking treatments' or therapies. Most psychiatrists are not trained as psychotherapists or psychoanalysts. You cannot become a psychiatrist at all unless you have first qualified as a doctor. From being a medical graduate it takes some seven years to become a psychiatric consultant.

Psychologists are specialists who do not need to have a medical degree. The science in which they do have a diploma or degree deals with 'the workings of the mind, especially in relation to behaviour'. Clinical psychologists first have a degree in psychology, then have also been trained to recognise and deal with emotional disorders. They cannot prescribe drugs but work through a variety of forms of psychotherapy. Psychologists who have a doctorate degree in their subject may use the title 'doctor', which can be confusing. A GP may refer his patients to a psychologist whose therapy he considers appropriate or whom his patient asks to see. Or the patients can make contact for themselves by phoning their District Health Authority, asking for the office of the District Psychologist (or equivalent), finding out what therapies they offer, and asking to be taken on.

Psychotherapists is a general name that describes the method of treatment used, not the qualifications of practitioners. A psychotherapist may be a psychiatrist, a psychologist, a qualified member of a particular school of psychotherapy, or have no specific training. The boundaries between psychotherapy, less well recognised forms of therapy, counselling, social work, self-help and support groups are not clear-cut. Most people who work solely as psychotherapists do so privately, though some are within the NHS.

Psychoanalysts have been trained in the particular type of psychotherapy called psychoanalysis. In-depth analysis is very intensive and lengthy (it can last for years) and is often confused with more generally used varieties of psychoanalytic psychotherapy. Properly speaking, psychoanalysts should have undergone at least a four-year training approved by the International Psycho-Analytical Association. Necessary previous qualifications include being medically qualified òr some equivalent qualification plus experience.

PSYCHIATRISTS

Most mothers who become seriously depressed or disturbed postnatally will see a psychiatrist. In *Depression: The Way Out of Your Prison* psychologist Dorothy Rowe describes the different ways in which they they may practise psychiatry. 'Now psychiatrists come in many shapes and forms. I can refer to them as "he" because there are in Britain few women psychiatrists, especially at consultant level. Each has his own idiosyncratic way of working, and so I can list only some of the varieties here. Some are wonderful – kind, understanding, sympathetic, wise, supportive and patient. Some are very strange, and leave you wondering who is the crazy one here. Some hold strictly to the medical model of depression and will give you pills and ECT and expect you to get better. Some try to give as little medication as possible and always have time to listen.

'Some visit their wards regularly and see their patients frequently while others make fleeting, irregular visits to the wards and appear to have abandoned their patients there. Some are trained therapists and some think psychotherapy is a waste of time. Some are skilled behaviour therapists while others think that if you reward a patient for anything you are only encouraging him to be manipulative and demanding. Some have a profound empathy with fellow human beings while others think that psychiatric patients are weak, inferior and stupid people. This last kind of psychiatrist often divides his patients into the "deserving" and the "undeserving" or frequently expounds his belief in "penis therapy", ie "All she needs is a good fuck" or "What he needs is a woman".'

Dr Vernon Coleman says, 'Current medical attitudes towards postnatal depression vary enormously from the sympathetic and useful to the primitive and potentially damaging. Most doctors deal with depression by attacking the brain rather than treating the mind.'

Very few mothers will be well enough informed, generally about psychological matters or specifically about the psychiatrists in their area, to be able to make a genuine choice about who they see. If they are admitted to hospital because of a crisis such as suicidal depression or puerperal psychosis they will have no choice. These circumstances inevitably lead to some mismatches of temperament and attitude between patient and psychiatrist. This compounds the problem of the professional being isolated from the patient by their training, and frequently by their sex, class, education and race. As a therapeutic relationship has to be based on trust and a feeling of safety, the sense of being interviewed by someone who is very much 'other' is a barrier to communication.

Ignorance of formal psychological concepts and terms may make a further barrier to an equal exchange, and the woman's unease may be increased by efforts to make her unformulated feelings fit into packaged explanations. If a woman is told by an 'expert' that she suffers from penis envy or has an unresolved complex about one of her parents she may remain unconvinced in her heart, but is unlikely to have alternative reasons to put forward for her distress. It will be impossible for professional help to reach a woman who feels mutinously that she is not depressed and guilty but has been as yet unable to work out that she is actually deeply, justifiably unhappy and terribly angry.

As there is such a wide range of psychiatric 'schools' a further mismatch between a particular woman's problem and her psychiatrist's way of working is possible. Psychiatry is deeply divided and ill-defined. 'There are critics of psychiatry who would not even call it a science at all, such is the uncertainty of much of the diagnosis and treatment. Indeed, one professor of psychiatry, Thomas Szasz, concluded that the only way of defining a mentally ill person was to say that it was someone who visited a psychiatrist,' says writer Jenny Pusey in *Here's Health*.

Individual psychiatrists may be sympathetic, understanding, compassionate and helpful, but many women feel (consciously or subconsciously) that the whole of psychiatry is couched in terms of 'patriarchal attitudes'. Some psychiatrists seem to assume that a woman who does not happily accept her male-defined role must be disturbed and need firm 'help' to make her happy (equals normal) again. This first implies that happiness, energetic enthusiasm and lack of confusion are the norm for all humanity, which they clearly are not. Then why only one half of the human race should be obliged to go around being little rays of sunshine all the time seems a question worth asking. Also, why should women be happy with a situation they do not like? Does not abnormality and sickness lie in *not* protesting?

Note the underlying assumptions in this description by a general practitioner (in *GP* magazine) of a visit. The patient 'to my "lay" eyes was mentally perturbed and very paranoid about her husband and her elder daughter. She was living in a chaotic state in her bedroom, which looked like a rubbish heap. She was not able to give the psychiatrist any adequate account of why the room was like it was.'

For years the GP had been admitting her to a mental hospital at regular intervals. 'Each episode had started in a similar fashion. Comments have been made that she was suspicious, obstinate, paranoid, verbally aggressive and unco-operative, and that she exhibited odd behaviour at home. Her attitude today was exactly the same as that described on her last admission two years ago – unco-operative, resentful, hostile and sarcastic. It was impossible to obtain any history from her. Not only had her pattern of symptoms been the same but her response to treatment has also been the same. Within a few days she became her normal, cheerful, happy self and ceased to display any paranoid ideas.' These expectations and attitudes recall the Stepford Wives syndrome (see Chapter 3) – 'do not make trouble or we will lock you up or otherwise do away with you'.

Being quiet and conforming are considered even more important than being cheerful, as is clearly demonstrated by the lack of attention received by those women who are sunk in despondency but do crawl around, performing their domestic duties adequately. There is a double-bind in thinking that allows this type of chronic depression in females to be viewed as a 'normal abnormality', hardly worth treating, certainly not worthy of the possibly lengthy and socially disruptive process of getting to the bottom of the problem.

Normality clearly means 'socially acceptable' not 'mentally healthy'. In *Women and the Psychiatric Paradox* Penfold and Walker say, 'There is apparent confusion in the psychiatric texts as to the definition of normality against which mental illness is to be judged. It is evident, in fact, that there is implicit agreement among professionals that what is normal is that which is socially acceptable as "that version of the world which has been sanctioned as reality." The dominant group in any society controls the meaning of what is valid information. For women and other subordinate groups, the version of the world which has been sanctioned as reality does not address

151

their lived experience; but because they have no accepted terms of their own, women have had few opportunities to understand this disjunction. The opportunities offered to them within the framework of the institution of psychiatry provide a way to experience the disjunction as proof of mental illness. That is, in some sense, its purpose: to present someone who has broken down under the strain of an intolerable existence, which must not be seen as intolerable, as someone to be "fixed up" with pills, treatment, and psychotherapy in order to go on living with the strains, or else as someone to be put away and cared for as incapable . . . "Train a person in psychological theory . . . and suddenly a world disastrously out of tune with human needs is explained as a state of mind." '

In the case of the new mother some psychiatrists see 'fixing up' a woman in terms of helping her 'to get back to her old self'. But after birth a woman is different and trying to return to her old persona and habits of life will create tension and illness, not cure it (see Chapter 7). Other psychiatrists think a mother needs help 'to adjust to her new role'. But they do not always mean adjust in the sense of work through a period of change and personal growth so that the woman becomes at ease with her extended, evolved persona. 'Adjust' can simply mean resume functioning as fast as possible with the minimum of disturbance to those around you. Back to the Stepford Wives.

While early experience clearly affects how anyone deals with the present, many women will be more concerned with the actualities of their current situation rather than hypothesised traumas and unresolved conflicts of early childhood. They may welcome deep insights, but feel it is more appropriate for them to work from the present backwards (when they have the time and emotional energy), than from the dim distant past forwards. Others may resent blame for their present distress being apportioned to their father or, more generally, mother, while difficulties relating to their present partner, their socioeconomic circumstances, and their role as women are brushed aside.

One enormous problem with any treatment by a psychiatrist is that, because of the tradition of dividing mind and body, it will almost certainly ignore possible physical causes or contributory factors. Some psychiatrists do concentrate on the chemistry of the brain and eschew psychotherapeutic techniques, but they do not consider the whole body in relation to emotional and mental states, although clearly there can be no mind as we know it without a body to house it, feed it, and express its workings. Whether there is a soul that can exist separately is another matter.

Because of this divided thinking there is a real danger that psychiatrists will completely fail to take into account the possibility of a bodily illness that is causing mental malfunctioning. For example, sustained stress, especially where there is sleep deprivation, predisposes to viral infections such as glandular fever or the more serious myalgic encephalomyelitis (see Chapter 4). One of the earliest symptoms of these infections is intense depression for no apparent reason. Other infections and illness can also produce mental symptoms. A paper written by Professor R C W Hall of the University of Texas and his colleagues describes how 100 psychiatric patients were evaluated for the presence of unrecognised medical illnesses. The results were that 46% were thought to have medical illnesses that directly caused or greatly exacerbated their symptoms and were consequently responsible for their admission.

In exploring the notion that PND might have physical causes several misconceptions are usually present – among those who are advocates for physical causes and those who cry 'not proven'. First is the idea that 'physical' means solely effects due to the action of sex hormones; second is the assumption that the balance of sex hormones goes awry in isolation and of its own perverse accord.

In considering the possible physical origins of PND, biochemical functioning has to be viewed as a whole – no one change occurs without involving a multitude of others (see Chapter 4). And the effects of stress must be looked at, caused by any one or any combination of the following: a difficult and unhappy birth, deep-seated psychological factors, social factors of all kinds, poor nutrition, the absorption of toxic elements, and sensitivity to a variety of foods and environmental chemicals.

It is obvious, yet again, that body and mind need to be considered as a whole. Fortunately, more doctors and a few psychiatrists and psychologists are doing this. Dr Stephen Davies says, 'It would be fair to say British research suggests that half our acute psychotic patients may be suffering from vitamin B1 and B6 deficiencies,' and believes that the assessment of psychiatric patients should include checking toxic metal poisoning, food intolerances and underlying physical illnesses but adds, 'psychosocial stresses do play a part.'

Dr Vicky Rippere, clinical psychologist at London's Maudesley Hospital, tries to help her patients by identifying allergies and by improving their nutrition. She does not use biochemical methods alone; once she has overcome these problems she goes on to use psychotherapy. Even psychotherapeutic techniques may work partly by biochemical means according to Dr Williams. Understanding and coming to terms with the source of their troubles calms an individual down. It 'may help to stabilise the internal chemical environment (eg by preventing the stirring up of unwanted hormones) and so may bring a measure of peace and tranquillity of mind.'

Hospitalisation

Sufferers from puerperal psychosis and some severe cases of neurotic depression may be admitted to a psychiatric ward or hospital. Reasons for admission are to supervise intensive treatment (through drugs, electroconvulsive therapy or psychotherapy), to take the mother away from stressful circumstances, to allow her a breathing space to work through what is happening to her, or to prevent her harming herself or her baby. It is now recognised that it is damaging to separate a mother from her baby and accommodation is usually for both, though the number of special mother and baby units is limited.

Some women regard hospital as a refuge, but many find a stay there frightening. The highly structured way of living takes away even petty control over their lives, there is loss of privacy and a few unofficial reports of sexual abuse by male staff. One woman recalls her stay in a psychiatric hospital. 'My lasting impressions are not happy ones. My feelings were extremely mixed. I remember the fear, panic and anger as the nature of my illness did not warrant my being kept in a psychiatric ward where there were patients with many different kinds of mental illness. Most of the patients frightened me, and some could become quite violent at times.'

Often there is no alternative to hospital admission because there is no one to be with the disturbed woman at home. A senior midwifery sister says that when faced with a severely depressed or outrightly psychotic mother she would usually try to get the mother's GP to admit her to a psychiatric hospital. Even if help were available at home she says, 'I don't know that when you have a really psychotic woman whether responsible mature female relatives round the clock could actually cope with a woman going through a psychotic crisis because they are so demanding and so divorced from reality but I think it would be incredibly hard.'

Chemotherapy

Psychiatrists' views on drugs vary. Some rely on them very heavily, some mix drug use with psychotherapy, some use minimal doses to lift a patient's spirits just enough for them to respond to other therapy, a few avoid drugs. As mentally ill patients exhibit measurable changes in their brain chemistry, it would seem logical to use chemicals to reverse these changes and improve the patient's mood. However, magic solutions to problems are rare and drugs do not take away mental disturbance, they merely stop the symptoms. Nor do they deal with what caused the original changes in brain chemistry. And psychotropic drugs have a lot of side-effects.

An additional worry for breastfeeding mothers is that drugs they take may enter their milk, yet 'statistical information on the range of drugs taken by mothers postpartum is virtually absent', according to an AIMS journal. Another danger in using drugs to treat mental illness is that they are a temptation to the suicidally depressed. Psychiatrist Colin Brewer points out that 'The rocketing suicide rate from prescribed sedatives and antidepressants ensured that by 1975 the overall suicide rate, which had levelled out [due to the introduction of non-poisonous North Sea gas], began to rise again . . . Suicide with psychotropic drugs far exceeds the incidence of suicide with aspirin.'

Hypnotics Adequate studies on milk concentrations of benzodiazepines used as sleeping tablets have not been done, yet in an in-patient survey of over 2000 mothers done at three Belfast maternity units 36% were receiving hypnotics.

Tranquillisers Barbiturates are seldom prescribed nowadays and tranquillising drugs are invariably benzodiazepines. As with the hypnotics, side-effects of these anxiolytics include drowsiness, dizziness, confusion, dry mouth, hypersensitive reaction, and a hangover feeling. Dr Coleman says firmly that 'benzodiazepines have no place in the treatment of postnatal depression', and many doctors do consider them inappropriate, but where anxiety is a strong symptom they may be prescribed. Their worst side-effect is addiction. Joan Jerome, founder of the self-help group Tranx, says 'We have, indeed, many, many people who have originally been prescribed [tranquillisers] for

PND, and by the time they have grandchildren they are still taking these pills!' Another complication of tranquilliser use is that they can release inhibitions, making it more likely that a mother could lose her temper and be violent to her baby. Then, as Dr Colin Brewer says, 'All tranquillisers work on the principle that if you're asleep you can't be miserable and if you're only half asleep maybe you'll only be half as miserable. The snag is that they do this by shutting down part of the brain and it is quite often a part that people need for coping with life's little problems. Is it really too shocking to propose that people should be encouraged to deal with the problems of existence by using all parts of their brain?'

Major tranquillisers These are often called anti-psychotic drugs. They can be used to treat mania and acute confusional states or, in small doses, for anxiety, tension and agitation. They are strong drugs with a range of unpleasant long-term side-effects.

Antidepressants There are two main groups of these drugs – MAOIs and tricyclics – plus some newly developed compounds that do not fit into either category. Monoamine oxidase inhibitors, says Professor Peter Parish in *Medicines*, 'block the breakdown (by the enzyme monoamine oxidase) of naturally occurring chemicals (amines) in the body. These amines (eg adrenaline, noradrenaline) are chemicals produced in response to emotion, fear and exercise and they have an effect upon mood – if they are high we may feel "high"; if they are low we may feel "low".' He also says, 'The adverse effects of MAOIs are greater and more serious than those of any other drug used in the treatment of psychological disorders.' Foods which contain tyramine (see Chapter 4) can interact with MAOIs to cause a sudden increase in blood pressure that can be fatal. Because of these dangers the use of MAOIs has greatly decreased. Most antidepressants given to women with PND are tricyclics. It is thought that they bring about an elevation in mood by producing an increase at nerve endings in the neurostransmitters noradrenaline and serotonin through blocking their too rapid re-uptake (see Chapter 4). They take two or three weeks to have an effect on mood but, says Malcolm Lader, professor of psychopharmacology at the London Institute of Psychiatry, 'The tricyclic antidepressants provide useful symptomatic relief in about four-fifths of depressed patients.' Tricyclics, by preventing reabsorption of the neurotransmitters into nerve terminals, deplete the cellular stores of neurotransmitters and interfere with proper brain function. Side-effects vary but include drowsiness, dry

156

mouth, blurred vision, nausea, constipation, urinary retention, tremor, rashes, sweating and loss of sexual desire.

There are some general problems associated with the routine use of drugs. Prescribed dosages do not usually take into account variations in patients' weight or metabolism, while Dr Brewer believes there are 'hardly any drugs for which there is a standard dose'. Nutritionists believe that most drugs aggravate the effects of nutritional deficiencies which can themselves cause mental problems. And when obvious mental symptoms that act as a warning disappear, the mother who was suffering from PND may be pronounced cured and be thrown straight back into her stressful life. Because there is still much healing still to be done, this may cause her to become ill again.

When it comes to claims for the benefits of drugs, the profit motive is always to be suspected. In a Standing Conference on Drug Abuse newsletter Syngen Brown of the Central Birmingham Health Authority warns, 'As the prescribing of benzodiazepine anxiolytics and hypnotics has now been restricted by the DHSS, advertising for these products is likely to become commercially unviable. It is reasonable to assume that the industry will respond to this situation by broadening the scope of indication for products which are not subject to the same restrictions. The most likely candidates for this response are the antidepressants. There is already an apparent increase in the promotion of these drugs as the "therapy of choice" for social problems ... The industry has demonstrated particular shrewdness by extending the scope of indication for these drugs to include states of anxiety and sleep disturbance. This "innovation" has been supported by expounding the view that depression is a frequent cause of anxiety and sleep problems. For as long as often misleading advertisements persist in their role of shaping the drug taking of the population there will be a continued increase in the problems associated with the medical use of psychotropic drugs.'

Electroconvulsive therapy

This is a highly controversial treatment which consists of passing an electric current through the front part of the brain. Electrodes are placed on the forehead and a low electric current is applied for a fraction of second. This produces a convulsion; to prevent injury a complete muscle relaxant is given and, to avoid panic, so is a quick-acting general anaesthetic. The seizure is followed by a coma lasting about five minutes, then an acute confusional state lasting an hour or more. There is a temporary loss of memory, particularly of recent events. There is a disagreement as to whether there is any permanent impairment of memory.

One mother who says she was 'not so much depressed as unhappy with my circumstances' describes the effects of her treatment. 'ECT affected my memory, but I forgot some of the pain, so I suppose it could be said I have been "cured" . . . The treatment blotted out the pain, but I also lost the intensity of the best moments of my life.' On the loss of memory associated with ECT the authors of *Dealing with Depression* (Nairne and Smith) say, 'It may well be important to you to retain your memory while trying to work out why you became so depressed.'

Whatever the price, and for reasons that no one as yet understands, the electric 'jolt' to the brain often seems to have an immediate effect on lifting someone's mood. This is one reason it is sometimes used in preference to drugs in treating PND. Antidepressants take two to three weeks to have an effect and a mother who apparently wants to kill herself and/or her baby is regarded as presenting a crisis situation that requires urgent action.

In the NCT booklet on PND one mother describes how ECT worked for her. 'ECT is absolutely painless. It worked instantaneously, completely alleviating my symptoms. For the first time in eight months I felt my old self. The only side-effects I had were a rather strange headache on treatment days, and an insignificant and temporary memory loss. I can't recall any of my husband's visits! I was in hospital for a month. Once home, I was gradually weaned off all the drugs and have felt very well since.'

Psychiatrists seem united in believing that ECT does no lasting damage. On 'unsubstantiated claims that ECT is not only ineffective but leads to permanent brain damage, I can categorically state that the latter is untrue,' says Professor Sydney Brandon in a MIND annual conference report. On the efficacy and superiority in the long-term of ECT, trial results have been conflicting and Professor Brandon goes on, 'it is imperative that this long-established treatment should be subjected to full scientific scrutiny, and if found wanting rejected.'

Dr Robert Palmer, senior lecturer in the department of psychiatry at Leicester University has an open mind about the use of drugs and ECT. He says in the same report, 'I detect at present an unhealthy polarisation between the biological and the psychosocial which is a powerful factor in promoting unproductive stereotypes and partial, prejudiced views.' He considers that ECT is probably used too much and certainly studied too little, and feels that, to date, 'trials have raised as many questions as they have answered'.

Many women patients and some doctors feel an instinctive revulsion at what appears a crude and barbaric practice and, as no one knows quite what ECT does to the brain, will not agree to its use. Some doctors feel extremely strongly about this form of therapy. Dr Coleman calls it 'a bizarre treatment' and says 'Anyone who treats depression with ECT needs medical help.'

ECT can be regarded as a life saver, an unwarranted assault on the brain, or a way of stunning women into compliance. Whichever it is it nevertheless shares with chemotherapy the disadvantage that, used on its own, it does nothing to help a woman discover why she has become disturbed, or see what she can do to change her attitudes or her life, and it may interfere with the slow processes of emotional and mental healing.

PSYCHOTHERAPISTS

The value of psychotherapeutic treatments in dealing with PND is disputed because they do not produce the quick, dramatic results of drugs and ECT. Often there is no one at home to care for a disturbed mother and her baby and getting the mother 'functioning' again becomes a priority.

Another problem is that, while pioneering psychiatrist Alfred Adler wrote that 50% of treatment consisted in the decision to seek help, most women who get PND do not themselves come to the conclusion that psychotherapy might answer their needs and make the first move. It is usually strongly put to them, by someone in the health service, that the time has come when some action must be taken. This element of pressure may undermine the effectiveness of therapy.

Although psychotherapy is probably of most value in preventing PND, or preventing a repeat bout, where the mother welcomes this form of help very limited therapeutic contact can produce remarkable changes in attitude and can take the heat out of an emergency.

Nairne and Smith say, 'In using a psychological approach we are able to look at depression as a state of mind and body which can result from a variety of life events and emotional dilemmas. Rather than understanding it as an illness that happens to someone out of the blue, we try to discover how a person becomes depressed through certain experiences and their reactions to these experiences.' Many mothers who have been 'cured' through drugs or ECT still find themselves asking 'why did I become ill?' and subsequent psychotherapy can provide some of the answers.

The description 'psychotherapist' covers anyone who helps those with emotional or mental problems through 'talking treatments'. The National Association for Mental Health (MIND) say, 'The aim of talking treatments is to help people gain an insight into the root cause of their distress, and to try and come to terms with the problems.' Some psychiatrists or GPs may use psychological therapy in conjunction with chemotherapy; some prescribe drugs while referring a patient elsewhere for psychotherapy. MIND say, 'Ideally there should be a range of treatments available so that the patient can find what works best for him, but in most areas this choice simply doesn't exist.'

The titles of psychotherapist and therapist are interchangeable. As all set out to promote healing of the mind, they could all claim they are entitled to call themselves psychotherapists, but it would be simpler for those seeking help if only people who had undertaken a specific training in psychotherapy used that title and everyone else kept to 'therapist'. To some extent this is, in practice, what happens.

The questions of what makes a competent therapist, how to protect the public from therapy that may be ineffective or harmful, plus what therapy to choose, have greatly exercised the professionals. Yet, according to Fraser Watts, head of the clinical psychology department at King's College Hospital in London, 'recent sophisticated surveys of research projects comparing various therapies have found no convincing overall differences in effectiveness.' From evidence he quotes it appears that experience, empathy, a caring attitude, objectivity, sensitivity, tact, warmth, genuineness, and respect for the client may be as or more important than theoretical understanding or technical competence. In addition, says Watts, 'There is something quite powerful about meeting regularly with a person who shows understanding and concern and who creates a belief in the possibility of change. This is something that nearly all therapies have in common . . . It looks as

160

though this non-specific aspect of being in therapy is often responsible for nearly all of the benefit the client gains.'

So, feeling that your therapist understands you and will listen sympathetically is, perhaps, more important than knowing anything about the type of therapy they practise. But, because therapists are trained not to make their ideas very obvious, a woman could be visiting someone whose philosophy about society and individuals, and particularly women, she disagrees with, or would disagree with if she sat down and thought about it. She may be being subtly indoctrinated without realising it. Because of this it is worth learning something about the basic types of therapy, and asking the therapist some direct questions on their views.

Therapy may be undertaken on a one-to-one basis, or may be group, marital or family therapy. The big division in schools of thought is between reconstructive therapies, which include all the psychoanalytic techniques, and therapies that are re-educative or supportive, the best known being behaviour therapy.

Psychoanalytic techniques

Freudian analysis is based on the recognition of unconscious mental processes, such as resistance, repression and transference, and of the importance of infantile experience as a determinant of adult behaviour. Through allowing people to talk freely while they listened, say the British Institute of Psycho-Analysis, 'Freud and his colleagues recognised that neurotic symptoms, such as phobias, obsessions, depressive ideas, inhibitions, perversions and even madness itself, seemed to be expressions of highly charged conflicting urges and dreads. Many aspects of these were outside the sufferer's awareness; they were unconscious. Thus it was realised that symptoms were not chance happenings; they were symbols of tortured states of mind . . .

'It was soon recognised that sufferers gained relief when they became aware of the hitherto unconscious emotional ideas that were expressed by symptoms. Thus the task of the psychoanalyst was, and is, not only to listen most carefully, but also to understand, from what is said and done in the sessions, the sufferer's underlying emotional conflicts of which she may have only a dim awareness. Communicating this understanding aims to help the sufferer gain a deepening and widening insight into her emotional life.'

Freud's ideas have given us enormous insight into previously mysterious workings of the mind. Unfortunately, 'reductive explanations tend to be historically specific' (Laura Chernaik). Sigmund Freud was very much a product of his nineteenth century, middle-class, Viennese, Jewish background and some of his explanations for mental processes and behaviour were far from eternal truths. It hardly seems fair to blame Freud for being what he was. The damage some of his ideas have done is to be blamed more on those followers who adhered rigidly to his work without attempting to separate out the historically specific elements. Those who used his work as a springboard have often been regarded as traitors, polluting the sacred word, instead of creative thinkers in their own right, although rival or derivative schools, such as that of Jung or Klein, established themselves firmly.

Many of Freud's theories grew out of his personal and cultural misogyny. From his writings and his work it seems he did not understand or, at heart, like women. His work enshrines the belief that women are less than men and inherently defective; that the only way they can be reasonably mentally healthy is to come to terms with their lot. To feminist Betty Friedan, Freudian thought has given a new life to old prejudices about women. In *The Feminine Mystique* she says, 'Without Freud's definition of the sexual nature of women to give the conventional image of feminity new authority, I do not think several generations of educated, spirited American women would have been so easily diverted from the dawning realisation of who they were and what they could be.'

However, this bias in the ideas of the creator of psychoanalysis does not negate the therapeutic properties of his techniques, nor mean that all who practise psychoanalysis proper, psychoanalytic or psychodynamic therapy adhere rigidly and blindly to the master's ideas in total. For example, some psychotherapists are more willing to view mental illness as a reasonable protest at an unreasonable world – or rather, protest at the lack of power a woman has to control the forces in that world that affect her. It is a matter of finding a therapist who is respectful, sympathetic and understanding to women in the role in which *they* see themselves or wish to achieve. A woman may feel at home with very traditional ideas, or she may feel negated by them.

Analytical psychotherapist Sheila Simmons says, 'Being a woman is very different from being a man. We live in totally different worlds.

Our emotional lives are better and fuller.' She has three sons and was involved in setting up the Birth Centre in London, dedicated to gentle birth, preferably at home, and has a particular empathy for mothers.

When a woman has a baby, says Sheila Simmons, 'For the first time in our lives there is something we can't run away from . . . There is no let up from the feelings which the baby arouses.' When a woman becomes disturbed postnatally 'What she desperately needs is a mother. She needs someone to hug her. She needs someone to understand and support her. A non-judgemental person to whom she can express her chaotic feelings that have welled up.'

She believes that the birth process can stir up long-hidden, buried emotional difficulties. On studies that dismiss birth itself as having any relevance to PND she says, 'These studies only look at people from the outside, not from the inside. They do not, for example, ask whether women who have psychotic episodes had unconscious difficulties in "letting the baby out" – these mothers could have been holding in all sorts of earlier disturbing emotional episodes.'

To Sheila Simmons healing works from the inside, out, 'from need, outwards, bringing to consciousness and dealing with those fears and ambivalent feelings which can inhibit our ability to give birth.' She thinks that because the intuitions and experience of women are disregarded, they feel a need for formal validation. Becoming a mother could supply that, but the new mother has no formal status and is rarely recognised, supported, praised.

Motherhood enables women to become mature, unlike men who can go on 'playing games' because they are never forced to cross a single divide and grow up. Problems women have with motherhood, or if the relationship with their partners is unsatisfactory and gives problems postnatally, can both be because a woman's emotional development has got stuck at some point. In exploring what is causing the block in development and how to loosen it, Sheila Simmons does not think in terms of induced guilt and a sense of unworthiness, but rather of anger and jealousy or envy. 'These are the two main things that come out, and women are not allowed to be either of these.'

As to avoiding PND, she believes psychotherapy before the birth might help. Because of the risk of finding the therapy disturbing before a stage of resolution is reached, it would seem best to explore any difficulties before planning a family, but Sheila Simmons thinks it could actually be good to start therapy, even once a woman was pregnant, although she would then go extra gently. She also feels 'it might help a woman to have a mother figure, someone with whom she had started a dialogue, there already,' before the birth.

Behaviour therapy

This form of therapy is most often given by psychologists, though it is employed by psychiatrists as well, and by psychiatric nurses. It originates in the principle of the conditioned reflex – habits of attitude and response to specific situations can be learned and therefore unlearned and replaced by other less destructive habits. Behavioural therapists concentrate on the present and the immediate future which appeals to those who feel delving around in the dim distant past is irrelevant. Behavioural approaches regard mental disturbances as the result of being insufficiently 'rewarded' emotionally for particular patterns of behaviour. By looking at the way a woman goes about her relationships and dealing with life, and proposing a more 'profitable' system that offers rewards, she is encouraged to change her life and live it in a way that does not cause her emotions and mind to protest.

Dr Victor Meyer, reader in clinical psychology at the department of psychiatry of the Middlesex Hospital in London, says, 'Some people have a resistance to behaviour therapy and call it a simplistic approach, a superficial approach or any other bad name they can think of! They assume that doing something in depth is always better than doing it superficially, but I wonder how many people can afford to operate like that. When one has a problem, one has to define the problem and describe it in such a way that there is a pragmatic way of dealing with it.'

Nairne and Smith say, 'This approach has something to offer, particularly if you are not very interested in exploring your "inner self". The danger might be that you could learn to cope better but avoid facing some more fundamental reason for your depression.' Behaviour therapy certainly may get quicker results in a crisis and be less disturbing than analytic techniques, but perhaps later on could be followed by more leisurely exploration of individual circumstances.

Counselling

There is really no clear distinction between psychotherapy and counselling, and counselling can have the status of a therapy in its own right. Counselling may cover individual psychological, sexual or psychosexual problems, or marital or family ones.

A general idea exists that counsellors give advice. Some may, if pressed to, but therapeutic counselling does not. Nairne and Smith say, 'The aim of a counsellor is to listen and try to understand what you are feeling and what you are trying to say. She will then feed back to you what she has heard in a way which shows that she has understood, without giving any judgements or advice. This is perhaps the best type of therapy for getting you through a crisis, when what you really need is emotional support rather than trying to understand yourself in more depth.'

Molly Ludlam of the Edinburgh Core Counselling Group describes counselling as 'a purposeful relationship in which one person helps another to help herself.' Mrs Susan Flint of the Samaritans organisation has dealt with desperate mothers and stresses the importance of being open to the person in distress and 'safe' to talk to. Giving time, she thinks, is the essence of successful counselling – 'time to listen in depth and particularly time to be silent.'

Because the needs of a dependent baby provide a pressure for a quick return to some level of normal functioning, counselling may be particularly appropriate for PND sufferers who are likely to be very vulnerable and in need of support and may initially be unable to cope with probing into themselves because of the overwhelming amount of pain that can then start to surface. The answer then is for the woman to seek a short-term solution and later, when she is ready, to start going into her deeper feelings – either on her own, using insights found during counselling, or with trained support.

Mind and body

Adjunctive therapies is the name sometimes given to those therapies that use physical expression – music, dance, drama. The body can give more accurate clues to what is going on in the mind than words. 'If a person comes to me for therapy and says they're feeling very depressed yet their movements clearly express pent up rage, then I'll

165

certainly believe their body,' says American dance therapist Kedzie Penfield. 'Dance is the most efficient way of communicating as it goes right back to the very beginning of our development in life,' says Jeanette McDonald who created the department of dance therapy at Langdon Hospital in Exeter. Dance psychotherapy can be traced partly to the mind/body growth therapies practised by Dr Wilhelm Reich, says Alix Kirsta in *Cosmopolitan*. 'Using movement either in conjuction with words, or on its own as a means of healing physical or psychic pain, marks the most recent development in the area of non-verbal "bodywork" systems such as Rolfing, Bioenergetics and the Alexander Technique.' Therapist Alexander Lowen says, 'Knowledge only becomes understanding when coupled with feeling. Since the mind has a directive function on the body, only a deep understanding coupled with feeling is capable of modifying structured patterns of behaviour.'

American humanistic psychotherapist and philosopher Eugene Gendlin held that psychotherapy produces change when people begin to feel preconceptual experiences with their bodies. A technique was devised to help raise the level of experiencing: 'Focusing consists of attending to the bodily felt sense of the problem and, without thinking in the usual way, waiting for the sense to explicate its own meaning.' Talking about psychosomatic medicine a group of Japanese doctors confirm that a high level of experiencing is essential to successful psychotherapy and draw attention to similarities between focusing and oriental thought, Zen in particular. 'Oriental thought has always valued not only the conceptual thoughts, but also the preconceptual sense . . . Holistic awareness or bodythinking which can occur under these levels of experiencing can be attained by learning techniques of bodily control and optimal functioning of the organism as a whole.' Body and mind serve and facilitate each other.

Which therapist?

Therapy is not necessarily a good idea and automatically helpful. Women need to be wary of authorities that define what women do or are as 'abnormal' without understanding what is normal. Diagnosis and 'treatment' can be used to patronise, disparage and control women, to remove them from the status of being fully adult human beings.

Visiting a therapist can also undermine a woman's trust in herself and in collective female experience. From Freud onwards women have been told they need professional help to interpret their experiences. Women could be wrong about their feelings and what they believe about themselves; they have no means of knowing either way. For a long time women have been told by middle-class white males what their feelings really are and should be. So they end up nervous, fearful, seeking validation, unable to trust their own judgement, as individuals or as a group. Psychoanalytic thought has traditionally given only a negative interpretation to early problems, stresses and traumas, when childhood difficulties can have a positive result, producing a woman who is wiser, stronger, with greater insight. When someone who has developed like this hits a problem patch, such as PND, her own processing of her childhood difficulties may be ignored or cast aside by a professional therapist.

Another kind of damage could result from psychotherapy. One woman with years of experience in dealing with new mothers believes reduction of external stress is critical and disapproves of psychological approaches. 'Rooting around in their pasts *causes* psychological problems. Psychotherapy is actually very damaging . . . Having psychological treatment is probably the most stressful event that can happen to any person.'

Clearly it is not possible to be blindly trusting about the benefits of psychotherapy in general, any particular technique or practitioner. Yet the therapist cannot reach or help a woman unless she trusts them. The only way out of this conflict is for a woman to have faith in her own reactions. If she does not like a therapist or feel comfortable with what they are doing she should leave. Even if the therapist is on the right track about the causes of her problem, they may be going at the wrong pace.

Most women, especially in a crisis, have limited or no choice as to what therapist they see – it is a matter of who is available nearby. However, it is worth specifying whether a man or woman is preferred. If a woman feels her therapist does not empathise with her, any 'treatment' will be wasted and she should ask for a change. If the relationship is moderately successful it could be a good idea to stick with the original therapist until the crisis is over, and seek another later when there is time to gather information and compare their ways of working and the opinions of women who have visited them.

It is worth asking for a therapist who is particularly interested in women's problems. Certain women therapists bring a 'feminist perspective' to their work while others offer 'feminist therapy'. Two women therapists who spoke to an NCT workshop about feminist therapy said they were attempting to integrate structured and feminist therapy by using two major principles – the personal and political, and viewing the therapist-client relationship in a more egalitarian light. The goals of feminist therapy they particularly aspired to were:

- To validate female experience, ie enable women to learn they are not crazy.
- Exploration of values and attitudes by therapist within an individual/family
- Attempt to keep the emphasis on change rather than adjustment
- Enhance the sense of personal power, ie encourage women to experience themselves as more self-directive, autonomous and more active.
- Encourage self-nurturance. Learn to value themselves and value other women as women. This can be a very difficult area as 'giving' is a status and some women may feel that something is being taken away from them when they are called on to put themselves first.
- Modelling by the therapist. Self-disclosure by the therapist can validate the woman's experience and widen her options.
- Enable women to express anger. Satisfactory resolution of feelings of anger is hard. All too often anger is converted into depression.

Some 10 years ago Luise Eichenbaum and Susie Orbach founded the London Women's Therapy Centre to provide therapy 'that addressed women's needs, understood women's experiences, and supported women's struggles'. Since then, 'women's therapy' has become more widely available, and local women's centres usually have the names of women therapists and counsellors (see Getting Help). Seeking therapy or counselling that is orientated to self-discovery and fulfilment, insight and strengthening, rather than 'adjustment' is probably the most productive course for most women.

IN THE FRONT LINE

Women with PND may be referred on to a psychiatrist or some form of psychotherapist, but who first notices that all is not well, or who does the mother decide to ask for help? Can those in the front line treat PND in their own right? And can they, through close contact with a mother, check an emerging episode of PND or even, by practices such as screening, prevent certain cases of PND altogether? Does the effectiveness of the helpers have as much to do with their personal qualities and the way they are organised as with particular professional qualifications?

Sympathetic research on mothers' problems has been carried out by Dr R Kumar and Kay Robson. One overall conclusion was, 'It is surprising how few childbearing women either seek or are detected as being in need of help for their emotional problems at a time when they are in repeated contact with the health services.' This could be because women do not realise how unwell they have become, because they do not think health professionals can help, or because they do not like or have confidence in the individuals they have dealt with locally.

One problem for a mother who might want to seek help is the variety of potential 'carers' she could come into contact with, ignorance about their training and roles, and confusion about how services are organised. Another barrier is that mothers are often unwilling to confide in someone in the context of a relationship they perceive as unequal. A third problem is that definitions of PND vary, there is fierce disagreement as to causes, and many carers see only what they have been taught to see, reflecting the limitations and prejudices of their training.

Midwives

In hospital postnatally a woman's distress may sometimes be noticed by her obstetrician but more often by a midwife who will have to decide what action to take – to help the mother herself or see that a psychiatrist, psychiatric nurse or obstetric and gynaecological social worker is alerted. Midwives are trained to pick up symptoms of PND of all forms, but they make up only 14–28% of postnatal ward staff and usually operate under strict guidelines as to how much discretion they have. Observations of a mother can be much more accurate and meaningful if a midwife knows her, if there has been continuity of care throughout the pregnancy, perhaps as far back as preconceptual counselling, and her contact is going to extend well into the postpartum period. Unfortunately such lengthy periods of care do not exist, but at least some efforts are being made to provide some contact antenatally, better co-ordination of care during the hospital stay and increased communication with mothers.

Midwifery sisters Jean Anne Ball and Jan Stanley are concerned about reducing stress in new mothers and have done research on the emotional needs of mothers postnatally. Their research, reported at a Royal College of Midwives conference, indicated that 'the way mid-wives provided care for mothers during the postnatal period had an effect upon transition to motherhood, and could, by increasing or decreasing stress in mothers, make a notable difference to the way each adapted to the demands of mothering her baby.' As a result a pattern of planned postnatal care was developed in their Mansfield hospital area. They had previously suggested that routine-based care had three main effects. 'It gave a false sense of security; the lack of flexibility militated against patient-centred care; it sapped initiative and critical appraisal of practice among midwives.'

Instead, the new care scheme involves discussion with each mother and liaison between staff. As a result 'The postnatal wards developed a more relaxed atmosphere than before . . . [They] have now been changed to combined ante and postnatal wards, and the midwives attached service the antenatal clinics, thereby making early contact with their prospective patients. In this way, the postnatal assessment is now built upon their antenatal plans under-taken in the clinic. Obviously this increases continuity of care throughout the mothers' involvement with the hospital and commu-nity staffs, and increases midwives' satisfaction.'

At the moment care is usually broken up so that different mid-wives (community or hospital based) see the mother at the antenatal clinic, during the birth and in the postnatal ward, while a community midwife may see her later at home. This division of care is, of course, avoided with home births. Provision of sensitive care in a hospital environment is very difficult because mothers are literally not 'at home'. Their emotional needs are not adequately met either. In one survey only 25 % of mothers said they were satisfied with their care and 25 % stated they were not satisfied. Ideally, 'a midwife should be a friend who helps the family deliver the baby and who helps the mother to care for her baby,' says Annie Wilton-Jones of the Centre for Advice on Natural Alternatives.

A hospital manager, Miss A Rider from St Helier Hospital, feels that hospital is not the best milieu for the postnatal period and that the midwife is not the main carer within the hospital environment. She would like to see postnatal care transferred into the community with the midwife as the responsible professional. Hospital stays average 5½–7 days, but most medical emergencies occur within 24 hours of birth and longer stays are unnecessarily disruptive. Ann Gee from Luton Hospital says, 'Mothers usually know best about when they should be discharged and [here] the midwife is given the responsibility for agreeing to or recommending discharge in most cases, not the medical staff.' Jane Paterson, a community midwife from Weston-super-Mare, points out that postnatal care at home is usually handed over to the health visitor at 10 days and wants to see community midwives caring for mothers for a longer time. Miss Paterson also makes a plea for carers to avoid complacency – she is concerned that if a mother comes home and seems to be coping, things are just left there.

Health visitors

These are members of the primary health care team. 'Her first job is to answer your questions – any questions, about anything,' say the NCT in *Pregnancy and Parenthood*. HVs work closely with GPs and run mother and baby clinics and, sometimes, weekly mother and baby groups. If an HV thinks a new mother is finding her situation overwhelming or is becoming disturbed she can inform the mother's GP, perhaps with a view to getting a referral to a psychiatrist. Or she can contact a social worker who can offer information about rights, benefits and practical help, or who may undertake various forms of therapy.

'Health visitors are trained nurses who have obtained a midwifery qualification or taken an approved course in obstetric nursing and have undertaken a year's practical and academic training in which the psychological aspects of childbearing are emphasised,' says Dr Kumar in *Motherhood and Mental Illness*. Because they must visit all mothers and their babies, health visitors have a unique role, but 'in most large cities, staff shortages dictate priorities and regular home visiting is exceptional. All mothers are seen at least once, but a single visit around the eleventh or twelfth day may not suffice for the detection of incipient puerperal mental disorder or of the risks of non-accidental injury. Postnatal depression and puerperal psychosis

171

can afflict women of all social backgrounds. Therefore, the presence of florid symptoms, and then only in the most disadvantaged women, may be picked up by the busy health visitor, who, incidentally, is not required to have any experience or training in psychiatric nursing.'

The Health Visitors' Association have called for the setting up of independent health visiting teams, freed from the governorship of GPs. HVA secretary Shirley Goodwin says that although 89% of HVs are attached to GPs' surgeries, 'GPs generally do not understand how to use health visitors,' and that GPs are mainly concerned with reacting to sick people while HVs are concerned with the prevention of illness and promotion of good health. This is as true of mental health as physical health, and independent status would increase the choice of how HVs dealt with disturbed mothers and so could increase their effectiveness.

Women's views of health visitors vary wildly. They are 'kind and intelligent' or 'useless'. They act as saviour in a crisis or their role is policing. 'They make sure you're treating the bairns right. Make sure your house is clean. Just like a spy, every six months or so. But you don't mind if they're OK.' If HVs are seen as an arm of authority mothers will not confide in them, and a valuable opportunity for picking up PND is lost. Single mothers can be particularly wary of professionals visiting their homes, fearing that if they are thought not to be coping this will be recorded in a file on them and could lead to their baby being taken away. Given the misleading comments that do end up in all kinds of files, and patients' limited rights of access to their own files, the fear has an understandable basis.

Shirley Goodwin says becoming a parent is one of the most stressful life changes yet, in her experience, new expectant parents have a mental block about the postnatal period. She considers that the HV can best help here by becoming a friendly and approachable figure antenatally, so that parents feel free to ask questions postnatally. To Ms Goodwin an HV can be many things. She can be a surrogate parent to the new parents themselves, an interpreter between them and the rest of the health service, a source of information and a figure of reliable continuity at a time of some uncertainty and confusion. But HVs need to give much less actual advice, and, rather, should help parents recognise the parenting skills they have. These skills are still intact, but deeply overlaid by a belief that 'the experts' know best. 'Fortunately the true experts realise that they do not.'

Lea Jamieson has worked as a parentcraft co-ordinator, training midwives and HVs. She feels they should examine their own level of maturity before trying to help parents who are going through experiences which require a high level of maturity if they are to be coped with successfully, namely birth and the adjustment to parenthood. Some HVs have found a way of breaking down barriers – running postnatal support groups. These enable mothers to gather practical information in a neutral environment, comments by HVs can be made generally and not personally, mothers can be made aware of what other services are available, and they can meet other mothers.

General practitioners

Most parents register their babies with their family doctors soon after returning home. Some mothers will return to the maternity hospital for a routine postnatal check-up at six weeks, but the majority go to their GP. According to psychophysiologist Ms Goudsmit, 'Several psychiatrists have remarked that the postnatal check-up at six weeks is a perfect opportunity to enquire how a woman is coping, whether she is unduly tired or anxious, if she is getting enough sleep and whether she is enjoying her baby.'

GPs are used to patients coming to them with vague problems, or physical symptoms that turn out to have emotional or mental origins, but women with PND do not automatically turn to GPs. In one study on psychiatric disorders of childbirth (Cox, Connor and Kendell 1982) it was found that 'The majority of women tried to continue with their household tasks and to meet their husbands' – as well as their babies' – demands.' And that 'although these women were distressed and bewildered by their inability to cope, they only rarely reported their depressed mood to their general practitioner.'

Again, it seems that postnatally disturbed women either do not generally appreciate the seriousness of their condition, or believe they have to find the solution for themselves. One factor holding mothers back from turning to their GPs could be that many are male. Or it may be that the six-week visit is badly timed for picking up the symptoms of PND – the blues are over and done with, psychosis is likely to have attracted attention earlier, maybe in the postnatal ward, and depression may only be recognisable later when it is well-established.

Liverpool GP Dr Katy Gardner says that GP postnatal care lags behind their antenatal services. She thinks the Royal College of General Practitioners should look at postnatal care because the six-week visit is often very variable and provides inadequate care. Problems like depression and psychosexual difficulties are often not picked up at six weeks. 'We need something else, perhaps at around three months, and we need to make it official.'

It has also been suggested that inadequate training is responsible for GPs' failing to pick up more than half those patients suffering from mental illness. Professor Michael Drury, president of the RCGP, says 'There is a low rate of initial pick-up, but many patients get diagnosed at a later stage. For instance, a depressive with anxiety symptoms may be treated for the symptoms before the GP is able to identify the causes.' He points out that GPs are still expected to concentrate on diagnosing organic diseases rather than mental illness, and that the cultural unacceptability of mental illness makes it difficult for both doctor and patient to accept a diagnosis of, say, depression. Yet GPs are in the front line of diagnosis and treatment of the mentally ill. Most depressed people see their family doctor and GPs refer very few of them on to a psychiatrist.

When faced with a woman who has PND her GP has the advantage of being able to assess the situation in the whole family. He can refer a patient to a psychiatrist or NHS psychotherapist, or suggest various forms of NHS, private or voluntary sector therapy – sometimes on a rather hit or miss basis. A unique service has been set up in London by two psychiatric social workers to fill the information gap. GPs and other health professionals can send their patients or clients to discover whether psychotherapy would help them and, if so, what form would be most suitable. This sort of service is needed nationwide.

If a GP wants to go on caring for a disturbed mother within their practice, they can do so by prescribing drugs – to help sleep or relieve depression. Some prescribe tranquillisers, though these are widely considered to be unsuitable for PND in addition to actually causing problems. Many GPs regard themselves as having an emotionally therapeutic role, while a few have undertaken psychotherapeutic training. Other GPs do not attempt to deal with patients' social, emotional and mental problems on their own but draw on co-workers attached to their practice.

Another GP in the practice may have psychotherapeutic interests that the woman's GP does not and they may suggest her seeing that doctor. Or use may be made of community psychiatric nurses who, in some districts, undertake patient assessment and aftercare in collaboration with GPs. Use may be made of nurse counsellors, although there is a great shortage of them. The educational charity Women's Health Concern has long advocated that nurse counsellors should work in doctors' surgeries. 'Worried women have always needed to talk to someone who will listen to what they have to say.' Social workers based at the Town Hall or psychiatric social workers with the health services may be brought in, or marriage guidance counsellors may be attached to a general practice.

The increasing importance of GPs' co-workers in dealing with PND is one aspect of a re-evaluation of how it is most advantageous to employ GPs' time – measured in hard cash and in the effectiveness of help offered. Most co-workers are women and their work is paid at a lower rate than that of doctors, so increased use of nurse practitioners, practice nurses and the like would make care cheaper, which should encourage the trend, if not necessarily for the right reasons. There has been a call for practice-based nurses to be available round the clock, with patients able to consult them directly without going through a GP, but the RCGP are against a radical expansion of the role of community and practice nurses and, in place of an overall national strategy, recommend that each practice decides for itself who does what. 'The nurse would work as a member of the team but she would remain accountable to the GP,' says their secretary Dr Bill Styles.

Midwives and nurses are currently demanding more responsibility, recognition and job-satisfaction. Increased use of nurses in the community will, almost inevitably, lead to an increase in their autonomy. 'The nurse who is just a doctor's assistant tends to see her work in terms of delegated tasks only and the value of nursing assessment is lost,' says nurse practitioner Barbara Stilwell. The Royal College of Nursing are pressing for nurses to have a wider role, and to be seen as equals with doctors. They say, to achieve full integration of nursing and medical services, family practitioner committees should be replaced by primary health care committees.

What would be the gains for women suffering from PND for various forms of nurses in the community having greater autonomy and being directly accessible? In a patient attitude survey in which Barbara Stilwell was involved several patients cited 'more time to discuss problems' as a reason for consulting a nurse practitioner. As nurses, midwives and health visitors are invariably women, and

175

social workers and counsellors are frequently female, mothers might feel more able to broach the subject of feeling depressed or disturbed postnatally with them. These workers are not seen to be as authoritarian or pressured as doctors, so mothers are likely to feel more relaxed and more entitled to ask for their time. Sympathy, understanding and advice based on firsthand experience can prove more therapeutic than any conventional, specialist treatment. 'The deepest need does seem to be for warm accepting human contact at this time,' says the NCT in *Pregnancy and Parenthood.*

PREVENTION

Mothers who have been through one episode of PND or are aware of the misery it can cause to their whole family want to find ways of avoiding PND completely, or at least dealing with it in its earliest stages. If PND is noticed early and help is available, the severity of the episode may be greatly reduced. Dr Dominian says, 'If puerperal depression is kept in mind, particularly by the health visitor, then an eminently treatable condition can be identified in time before it causes utter havoc to the marriage.' Whatever the treatment it is 'even more important the couple should have the condition explained to them. This will lift an enormous amount of self criticism and guilt on the part of the wife, who is utterly perplexed by her state. The husband's support and availability need to be mobilised. Advice should be offered on the practical side of running the home and looking after the baby in a way that the mother can have time and rest for herself. If necessary and possible help should be obtained. The relatives should also be informed so that they can provide extra support.' Dr John Cox cautions, 'Reassurance that recovery is rapid or that the cause is hormonal is not always wise because difficult family relationships may not then be discussed.'

Whether PND is picked up in its earliest days depends largely on the efficiency and awareness of the community health services in any given locality. In Britain the situation is highly variable, depending on local priorities. The Maternity Alliance say, 'there is increasing recognition that the provision of postnatal services is failing to match needs, particularly in relation to care of the mother . . .' They are pressing for changes such as reorganisation, more independence and information for health visitors, community midwives and nurses, and more convenient clinic times.

The way support services deal with the mother is all important if valuable opportunities for recognition of PND and early help are not to be lost. Practical, general, and non-directive advice seems the most effective, and the closer and more familiar the health professionals are to the mother, the better. Avoiding 'them and us' divisions is critical in establishing the mother's confidence in local services. The local health centre, clinic or doctor's surgery should feel to a mother like her place as much as 'their's'.

Mothers can be reached by printed information on PND but, judging by the tone of the limited amount available, the authors are frequently out of touch and limited by preconceived notions. Leaflets and brief mentions in books are mostly extremely vague and either take the line that PND is near inevitable but not very important or are full of bland reassurances that imply recognition equals a near-instant total cure. 'Postnatal depression is not usually a physical illness. It is easily understandable, and nearly as easily curable, using the right tools,' say the authors of *Pregnancy and Birth* (Macy and Falkner) optimistically.

The practical and day-to-day advice offered is often alienating in its lack of realism ('always indulge yourself daily with half an hour in the bath' or 'get more rest'), and can be harmful. Telling a possibly breastfeeding woman to diet to get her figure back in order to ensure her husband's continued interest is insulting to both men and women, shows a repugnant sense of values, and is likely to cause depression and reduce the mother's milk supply. Self-help support groups often provide much more useful advice in a more understanding tone (see Chapter 6).

Is a reduction in the number of cases of PND best achieved by the preparation of all couples for parenthood or by screening out 'vulnerable' mothers and concentrating help on them? No one knows how to prevent PND, so all preventative measures are safety nets with very large holes. 'The only certain way of avoiding puerperal depression is by avoiding pregnancy,' says Dr Brice Pitt realistically. So called preventive programmes involve establishing which mothers might be at risk, evaluating all their circumstances, giving them advice on avoiding those stresses known to predispose to PND, and watching them carefully after the birth. Dr Brice Pitt in *'Partners in Care': Puerperal Depression* suggests the following measures to help a woman.

- Careful appraisal of her personality, family and past history, reaction to previous childbirth, present social circumstances, marriage, state of mind, attitude to present pregnancy and any special problems.
- Arranging extra support where indicated from within the family, by a social worker, midwife or other clinic staff, general practitioner or sometimes psychiatrist. Try to see that after the birth the mother will have little more to cope with than her baby.
- Antenatal counselling should allow the expression of fears and negative feelings, provide education in the manifestations of depression so that help is sought soon, indicate informal as well as professional sources of help (eg other new parents), give advice to reduce rather than take on responsibilities, recommend avoiding moving house soon before or after the birth, and involve the husband fully.
- Vigilance for early signs of mental disorder enables it to be treated promptly.

The importance to lessening the chances of PND of involving the woman's partner is often overlooked (see Chapter 6). In *Transition to Parenthood* the Thomas Coram Research Unit say, 'Fathers generally had little dealing with the [maternity] services. Antenatally they were specifically excluded by hospital policy from attending the clinic or the [ultrasound] scan; during the inpatient stay they were excluded from taking any part in the care of their baby; daytime visiting largely prevented contact between fathers and health visitors, except in the week or so after hospital discharge which most fathers took off work. Few fathers visited child welfare clinics.' When men have been excluded in these ways they may become increasingly isolated from their partners throughout pregnancy – which in itself could cause a mother to become depressed. Then, if she does suffer from PND, a man may be too out of touch to reach her and help her, or he may deliberately withdraw, feeling resentful and unsympathetic to her problems.

A programme aimed not at prevention but at early detection of postnatal depression could be carried out by GPs or health visitors, using a new rapid screening questionnaire. The Edinburgh Postnatal Depression Scale (EPDS) was devised by Dr John Cox, J M Holden and R Sagovsky at Edinburgh University's department of psychiatry. The EPDS can be used routinely to screen all mothers at six to eight weeks postnatally. The GP's postnatal checkup, a home visit or child health clinic visit are regarded as suitable opportunities for completing the scale, which the mother does herself. The questionnaire consists of 10 questions, each with a choice of four responses, and a simple scoring the level of which indicates those mothers who are 'likely to be suffering from a depressive illness of varying severity.' The authors stipulate 'the EPDS score should not over-ride clinical judgement. A careful clinical assessment should be carried out to confirm the diagnosis.'

The test is extremely quick and simple for the mother to complete, and a health professional to evaluate the score, and trials have shown it can pick up more than 80% of women with PND. The EPDS must seem a valuable tool to busy health professionals, but mothers may find it threatening, feeling that filling in the form truthfully could result in their being labelled a failure, a problem, ill, unsuited to being in charge of their baby, or 'a suitable case for treatment'. A woman might be angry or unco-operative, feeling she was being asked to pass one more test as a mother.

Like all diagnostic tools it could be abused. It encourages professionals, yet again, to assign people to ready-made categories and not to trust their own judgement – about the individual in front of them, or the validity of such categories at all. For the mother, it means that she does not choose to come forward for help – and she may have valid reasons for not wanting to – but her secrets are winkled out for her own good, and someone else makes the decision that she ought to be helped. Depending on the professional background and personal experience of the assessor, the help she is offered may be limited and unsuitable. For example, certain GPs will offer drugs but no therapy or support.

Diagnosis implies treatment. A woman who knows that she is miserable but is still busy working out why, and disapproves of the treatment offered, risks being labelled difficult and unco-operative if she refuses – something she would have avoided if she had quietly concealed her problem until she was ready to confide it and had found someone she wanted to confide in. As diagnosis through such a simple test could become production line, there is a risk that treatment could be seen as equally straightforward and amount to little more than an attempt to swiftly remove the symptoms without considering why they were there – perhaps suppressing a sane response to an insane situation.

Organising measures aimed at avoiding PND or picking it up early requires commitment, planning and finances. But the lack of preventative facilities is not just due to administrative problems. There are practical difficulties to overcome and ethical issues to take into account. Acting to cure something presumes you know what causes it. With PND the most dedicated professionals disagree vehemently or have to state with due humility that they still do not know for sure. Preventative schemes would be hampered by lack of knowledge.

Another aspect is that such state-organised forward-planning, linked to reproduction, has Big Brother overtones to many. Certainly pregnant women, in their concern for their babies and for their own safety, are very vulnerable to indoctrination. With the best of intentions and the kindliest of attitudes it is possible for screening schemes, counselling, therapy and psychotherapy to perpetuate the situations – with regard to women's roles, their relationships with men, and the social background – that may have caused or contributed to PND in the first place.

Views on prevention will be limited by views on the cause of PND – a truly composite approach to each case is rare. For example, nothing in body or mind works in isolation but the roles of general nutrition, specific nutritional supplementation, excluding environmental chemicals, and hormonal treatment in preventing PND are usually ignored, although their degree of success would probably be the easiest to evaluate (see Chapter 4).

Specific psychotherapeutic preparation of chosen mothers has been condemned as 'useless, harmful and arrogant' and a 'very dangerous digging and trawling around in the mind'. General counselling on parenthood may fail because couples resist knowledge that would upset their ideas. And all who attempt to teach preparation for parenthood – practical or emotional – during pregnancy run into a blank on the part of parents in seeing past the birth itself. Thomas Coram found that only a third of mothers felt they have been adequately prepared for parenthood. But, 'Most mothers who felt inadequately prepared also believed that nothing could have been done to make them more so: many felt that the experience was so personal, so unpredictable and so overshadowed in pregnancy by the prospect of the birth itself, that helping prospective parents anticipate the early months of parenthood would be difficult or impossible.'

It seems likely that practical preparation for parenthood and the field of individual growth would be better dealt with separately; and both, ideally, need working on before a family is started – before, perhaps a stable relationship can be founded? Broad-based developmental help, offered to all individuals, rather than narrowly-based programmes, directed at mothers chosen because they were thought to be at risk of PND, might result in fewer problems for new parents (and their children) generally. And this approach would avoid the necessity of making value judgements and the problems of labelling women.

For the present, programmes aimed at preventing PND might be less intimidating and encourage mothers to be more open if they avoided operating through figures in authority evaluating women's chances of succumbing to PND. Instead, they could offer women information that made them aware of the existence of PND in all its forms, what is thought to increase or decrease the likelihood of it occurring, and what support networks are available. This would give all but the most severely disturbed mothers the opportunity to decide for themselves if something was wrong and who they wished to discuss this with.

CARING SCHEMES

Concerted efforts to reduce the incidence and effects of PND, through identifying in pregnancy mothers at risk, early postnatal diagnosis, support and treatment are rare, but a few good schemes do exist whose examples could well be followed. They are characterised by an open-minded, flexible and individual approach, have developed organically round women's needs, and offer sympathy and warmth above all but, beyond that, they operate differently. These are some ways in which it would be possible to help mothers, if more schemes were set up.

Obstetric liaison service

Such a service, based on two hospitals in the Aylesbury district, is run by psychiatrist Dr Diana Riley. It deals with postnatal depression and puerperal psychosis and grew from her special responsibility for pregnancy-related psychiatric disorder. Dr Riley believes that they 'must deal with every woman individually' and after birth there is a great need for 'rest, peace, care, support, pampering, nurturance, mothering.'

Referrals to her outpatient clinics came first from GPs and other psychiatrists. Dr Riley says, 'Increasingly, however, patients thought to be "at risk" for the development of postnatal psychiatric illness have been identified in the antenatal clinics and referred early in pregnancy. This allows me to gain a knowledge of the patient and her social circumstances before delivery, giving a baseline against which to monitor her progress in the puerperium. It also offers the possibility of providing antenatal treatment, reassurance and practical help where necessary.' The average time between referrals (both ante and postnatal) and first appointments is 10 days, while in the postnatal wards mothers are usually seen within 24 hours.

The service has an admission rate of 1.76% for postnatal depression (against a general incidence of 10–15%), so 'It is obvious that the vast majority of cases are either unrecognised or are being adequately treated by general practitioners.' On the quantification of PND Dr Riley says, 'Many of the standard symptoms of depression . . . are confused by the postnatal state. In particular, the existence of physical discomfort and changed social circumstances may make the differentation of clinical depression from unhappiness very difficult.' One standard questionnaire she has found useful gives 'not only a measure of depression but also of outwardly directed irritability; an important factor to take into account when the mother's ability to care for her baby is in question.'

Only a very small number of women get puerperal psychosis. Dr Riley believes they fall into two groups. One has a history of mental breakdown, even schizophrenia: presumably there is a hereditary predisposition in this group. The other, where a woman is competent, healthy, balanced, happy, with no childhood problems, but suddenly becomes very disturbed, seems to have hormonal imbalances postnatally. Before the service started the number of admissions for postpartum psychosis in the Aylesbury district was two and a half times greater than it is now. 'It would be encouraging to suppose that antenatal intervention is having some beneficial effect,' says Dr Riley.

Some disturbed women need to be admitted and finding suitable accommodation for mothers with their babies was a problem at first. One reason was 'some women found it unacceptable to be admitted to part of a large district psychiatric hospital containing long-stay patients. In their depressed state it was all too easy for them to feel that they might have a chronic illness.' Now one hospital has a self-contained unit in an adapted flat. With voluntary funding for the decorations and furnishing 'every effort has been made to make it cosy and homelike'.

Much of the admission time is actually 'spent out of hospital, either with relatives or at home with suitable supervision from community psychiatric nurses and family aides, with regular review from the hospital team. Patients are only officially discharged when all those involved are satisfied they are coping well with their babies and domestic responsibilities. Our low readmission rate reflects this caution . . . It is very clear that the amount of time spent in hospital often relates more to social circumstances rather than severity of illness. For example, experience has shown that even moderately severe hypomania can be managed very well at home when a relative is able to be with the patient full-time.'

Mild postnatal depressive illness, especially in women reporting other hormonally induced mood changes such as depression on the contraceptive pill or premenstrual syndrome, appears to respond to treatment with vitamin B6 (pyriodoxine) alone, usually 100mg daily (see Chapter 4). Some women need other medication. Dr Riley feels that low doses of drugs with a limited period of prescription are helpful to get a woman well enough to make the changes in her life that depression signals are needed. 'She can't do it all by herself at that initial stage.'

In choosing an antidepressant, 'The choice for this group of patients is not an easy one. Since the majority complain of excessive tiredness, they are unwilling to tolerate the added soporific effects of medication. All drugs in the tricyclic group produce sedation . . . The tetracyclic group of drugs are relatively ineffective . . . Particular care is taken with breastfeeding patients to keep the dosage as low as possible, and to time medication so as to minimise the amount transferred in breast milk . . . The minor tranquillisers, especially benzodiazepines, are avoided.'

Treatment other than medication is also employed, by itself or in combination. Apart from therapeutic interventions in the clinics, weekly individual psychotherapy, relaxation training and behavioural programmes are used. In counselling, Dr Riley will ask the mother's partner in to explain that for a woman to be free to become more herself, do things that are interesting and have less domestic grind, will mean changes in the home and relationship.

Dr Riley uses crisis methods – drugs and occasionally ECT – when women come to her when deep into a depression. To avoid this, an early pick-up is very important. If a woman has had PND once, there is a 75% chance of recurrence and 'we must help these women'. Where women are referred to the service during pregnancy because of previous psychiatric illness, postpartum recurrence rates are rewardingly low.

Awareness on the part of the mother is a great help. While recognising that the possibility of PND, stillbirth and neonatal death or handicap are tricky subjects to introduce at antenatal classes, Dr Riley says, 'Many mothers have expressed a wish that these matters should be dealt with at some stage, preferably at a joint meeting with the prospective fathers, so that families are at least aware that childbirth is occasionally less than ecstatic, and early symptoms of psychiatric disorder can be reported, knowing that interest and help is available.'

With regard to staff involvement, contact with the midwifery school 'provides an opportunity to explore the feelings of midwives and to look at their role as facilitators of a major life event in a family rather than as ministrators to sick patients.' Regular meetings and discussions take place with health visitors and district community midwives. Where attendance at clinics is difficult community psychiatric nurses provide regular support, supervision of medication and progress, and liaison with Dr Riley. Self-help groups in the community (see Chapter 6) have been utilised both to bring the service to the attention of women in whom they recognise early symptoms, and to support and counsel patients and ex-patients.

The hospital nursing staff have played a key role. 'Their high standard of psychiatric nursing skills has been more than matched by the tender loving care which they have provided for the patients, their babies and families . . . visiting hours have been flexible to say the least. Nurses have spent much time in psychotherapeutic interventions with patients and with relatives, particularly husbands, helping them to support their wives and to understand more about their illness . . . Ward staff have visited patients in their own homes; patients have attended the ward on an informal daycare basis, and frequently return to make social visits. It has often seemed that the presence of a baby on the ward has enhanced feelings of mutual concern amongst patients and staff, and has led to a more optimistic atmosphere.'

On staffing generally, Dr Riley says, 'The success or otherwise of the obstetric liaison service depends above all else on the commitment and expertise of the personnel involved. Thus it is important to have continuity of care and a team of workers in close co-operation.' Maturity and special qualities are called for. 'The nursing staff need to be those particularly interested in this work. As with child psychiatry, dealing with mother and baby relationships can awaken primitive and often hostile feelings in those whose own experience of mothering has been less than satisfactory ... The staff need to be quite exceptional, not only experienced in handling babies and in recognising fluctuating levels of psychiatric disturbance, but skilled in allowing the bonding process to develop at a rate acceptable to a disturbed mother, and in being able to "mother" the mother herself without interference with her autonomy.'

The need for the service is clear. 'Postnatal illness represents a substantial demand on psychiatric services, and an even greater degree of morbidity in the community which may perpetuate itself into succeeding generations.' Dr Riley sums up the value of the service's work. 'I have no doubt that referral during pregnancy of those women thought to be vulnerable to postnatal psychiatric disorder is helpful in prevention. Quite apart from any treatment that may be offered, it is often therapeutic to be able to discuss fears about labour and the puerperium with someone not actually involved with the delivery. Practical help can also be arranged, social problems discussed, and antenatal counselling provided for those with longstanding neurotic disorders.'

Postnatal mental illness unit

Psychiatrist Dr Margaret Oates runs a unit for disturbed and depressed new mothers at the Queen's Medical Centre, Nottingham. She says, 'I feel very strongly that women who become mentally ill in relation to childbirth, or who develop conditions of personal distress, psychological or mothering problems, both need and require a special service. I think that this need is not based on the uniqueness of their illness, but rather that their conflicts, the reality of their situation and the presence of small babies, demands that the service should operate in a different way for this particular group of consumers, and should be run by a group of people who are empathic and sensitive to the needs of women with young children.

'I also feel very strongly that until recently, women who developed mental illness in relation to childbirth, be it of major or minor kind, have too often been deviantly labelled as rejecting their feminine or mothering roles, and have too often been categorised as incompetent and bad mothers. The romantic myths of motherhood are all pervasive, particularly amongst the medical profession, and one of the things that a service such as ours has to offer our patients is a more realistic understanding of the realities of both being a mother, and also of being a small child.

'Almost by definition, we spend most of our time dealing with very seriously ill women, and relatively little with the more common and problematical areas of postnatal depression that are largely dealt with by consumer groups, self-help groups and health visitors. For the very seriously ill women our priorities are that treatment of her illness should not involve separation from the baby. It is our proud boast that in Nottingham no woman needs to be hospitalised without her baby within a year of childbirth if her mental state requires admission to a psychiatric unit. In other words, we offer mother and baby admission as a routine.

'Our second priority is to achieve by whatever means possible, the most rapid resolution of her mental state, and to, from a very early stage of her treatment, maintain the mother/infant dyad, therefore accelerating her return to normal functioning and avoiding the guilt and alienation that women often feel towards their babies if their treatment has excluded them from their baby. We also spend quite a lot of time liaising with the obstetric service and see women during pregnancy who have had past histories of mental illness in relation to childbirth, and engage both the patient and the obstetrician in various strategies that might reduce risk, or at the very least, involve early detection and rapid treatment if such an illness should recur.'

Postnatal project

This scheme in Lewisham, south east London, is aimed at the prevention or early recognition of postnatal depression (the blues and puerperal psychosis are outside its scope). It is funded by a trust as 'a pilot study of an intervention programme to reduce the prevalence of postnatal depression in an inner city area'. Research psychologist Dr Sandra Elliott, psychiatry registrar Tessa Leverton and liaison health visitor Marion Sanjack are responsible for running and developing the programme.

The project aims to reach mothers through a series of monthly group meetings, held from the time the women are about four months pregnant to six months after their babies are born. If the research confirms the value of this approach, similar classes could be provided as a routine part of the antenatal system, run by health visitors and/or midwives, backed up by psychological and other services where individual referral or consultation for advice was required.

Having decided that an educational package is what the majority of mothers would expect, want, and respond to, further decisions were made about how to put this across. Group sessions make more economical use of limited resources, they are in tune with the less threatening presentation as education not therapy, and they offer a chance for mothers to meet and support each other. Individual counselling is offered as a back-up. Numbers of 10–15 are enough to keep a group lively but not so many as to be overwhelming.

The atmosphere is kept warm and informal by rejecting a lecture format, arranging the chairs in a circle and providing refreshments. Meetings early in the programme are structured for most of the session, with the proportion of open discussion time increasing up till the last pregnancy meeting and postnatal meetings which have no formal structure. One important aspect of the project is that mothers are encouraged to seek help or advice on an individual basis when they feel they need it. Each woman is given a telephone number and two times during the week when they can phone, both by her community health visitor and her group leader.

The project works through providing certain elements:

Professional contacts Community health visitors normally meet a mother late in pregnancy. In the project they make an additional visit to mothers in early pregnancy. Contact with group leaders is maintained through pregnancy and the postnatal period.

Social contacts Emphasis is placed on establishing relationships with other young mothers, both inside and outside the groups. One study (Graham and McKee 1980) found that at one month after the birth 25% of their sample reported having no contact with other mothers; of these, 60% said they would appreciate such contact.

Knowledge about PND This prepares parents for the possibility of experiencing negative emotions after birth, teaches them how to recognise PND, and encourages them to seek professional or other help promptly.

Knowledge about children The leader encourages realistic expectations about early motherhood and early child development.

Ideas on parenting The object is both to provoke thought about changes in life style that may occur so that appropriate plans can be made and to provide suggestions for consideration, such as welcoming suitable help.

Factual information A list of relevant organisations, parenthood manuals, and recommendations on children's play materials and books are provided.

'Throughout the programme of group meetings,' says Dr Elliott, 'the aim is to encourage discussion on a variety of issues and to allow each woman to consider a range of possibilities. A non-directive style is adopted by the leaders who do not describe how parenting will or should be but how it may be and the choices available.'

One important effect of pointing out the possibility of having negative emotions after birth is that this gives mothers 'permission' to experience and express these emotions without guilt and feelings of failure. Lack of opportunity to express negative emotions about their children, or guilt about these feelings, increases stress, in some cases leading to clinical depression. Accepting that one is finding it hard, feeling low and tired and so on, without feeling guilty may be the start of recovery. Painting a realistic picture of motherhood helps to balance the idealisation and romanticisation of the state that makes women feel failures if they find it boring or difficult, then guilty because they are failures, plus helpless to improve life.

Dr Elliott feels that services for pregnant women and mothers of young children need to be developed in all areas, not just the health service. She feels the aims of changes should be to:

- produce better preparation for parenting
- remove unnecessary stress, including isolation
- provide support and help mothers to understand it is legitimate for them to seek it
- acknowledge the value of the mother's role
- make access to professional and personal help easier and possible without requiring a 'label'

If, through attending the group sessions, mothers come to realise that the job of mothering is difficult and valuable, they will appreciate why they feel stressed and have a sense of self-worth to sustain them. Whereas, 'If a woman fails to recognise that there are times when a mother's job can be ranked amongst the most stressful occupations, then she will make inappropriate attributions for any difficulty in coping, irritability, lack of energy or low mood that she experiences.'

The significance of the widespread lack of acknowledgement of the potential stresses in a mother's role is that 'it leads to the failure of people round her to offer appropriate instrumental, emotional and self-esteem supports and leads the mother to attribute her difficulties to personal inadequacies rather than to the stresses inherent in her situation.'

Dr Elliott says the traditional system of care 'often leads to women struggling alone with stress and depression or using various "tickets" to professional help. Such tickets include complaining about her baby's health or behaviour,or her own physical health, to the GP, or about housing problems to a social worker, or labelling herself as unable to cope with the "simple" job of being a housewife and mother to the health visitor or, indeed, using the label "postnatal depression".'

Through the Postnatal Project 'Women are encouraged to recognise the value of their abilities to cope with the stresses of motherhood and also their right to help in coping with these stresses.' If a mother does become depressed Dr Elliott encourages her to seek professional help as soon as possible since, 'the less time a woman suffers alone and unsupported during depression the better.'

Home-visiting and befriending scheme

The co-ordinator of the charitably funded New Parent Infant Network (Newpin) is Anne Jenkins, a former local health visitor with marriage guidance training. She sees postnatal depression as part of a wider problem. 'Although we have a comprehensive health and welfare service throughout Britain, in the main we have lost the ability to view people as unique and therefore underestimate their individual needs. This disenchantment with the system, the disquieting soaring child abuse figures, the amount of depression, particularly amongst young mothers, and the increased isolation, led me to look at ways in which changes could be brought about to make for a more healthy and stable society.' Newpin operates in Walworth, south London, a typically deprived inner city area, but the way in which it helps women to help each other and themselves could apply to mothers anywhere.

Newpin has a few professional staff, fulltime and part-time but the main work of supporting depressed mothers is done by other mothers. The scheme 'concentrates on offering an emotionally secure, loving and caring environment alongside the expectation, whether sooner or later, to take in some measure, control of one's own life.' It is 'a group of individuals working together to improve the quality of life for themselves and their children, and by a process of self-learning, recognise the value of creating good relationships both personally and in the wider sense of community.' Depression, isolation and difficulties with parenting are the major problems of women who use Newpin and are most suited to its approach, which aims to raise the self-esteem of mothers and the quality of life for the whole family, rather than to treat specific problems in isolation.

A most important aspect of Newpin is the premises. 'I cannot overestimate the advantages of having a centre which is available to mothers and their children . . . having a base where difficulties of managing oneself and one's life can be expressed does enable problems to be contained and controlled,' says Anne Jenkins. The property is comfortable and homey, with a living room, playroom and kitchen, and open during the working week so that anyone using the centre can drop in whenever they want or need to.

As to those who use the centre, 'The only criteria for involvement with Newpin is that people are mothers or the main carers of children.' Supporters and supported overlap. 'If you ask me how I decide, I would have to say that I see growth potential in everybody, but in some it is at a quicker rate than others.' Supporters volunteer and are trained in the centre. 'One of the effects of training is to immediately raise the level of how mothers see their own status . . . even though the potential for supporting may not be possible for some time, nobody who has previously been a referred mother is denied training.'

The preparation course is set up 'to allow free expression in order to create a feeling of non-judgement and toleration' and intended to create an awareness of self and others. It lasts for 18 weeks of twice-weekly morning sessions. One morning is spent on talks and discussions on personal health and well-being, pregnancy and birth, understanding childhood and children's needs, personal and social stress, and attempting to make some sense of their own community.

The other morning is spent with a trained counsellor skilled in group work who facilitates personal understanding and awareness of the perplexities of human relationships, which in turn engineers a feeling of trust and respect. 'For many of the mothers, this may be the first time they have experienced these feelings in their lives.' Because of the demands of the befriending relationship, and because the supporter mother herself is often vulnerable, all support mothers attend a weekly closed group where they can discuss personal difficulties or those they may encounter with their referred mothers.

Mothers may be referred to Newpin formally by health visitors, social workers and GPs, or informally by other mothers. No mothers are seen unless they have expressed a wish to become involved. This 'gives an opportunity for decision taking and personal responsibility which is a crucial step.' Support takes place through home visiting by a befriending mother and, once she is ready, being invited to drop in to the centre in her company, plus, where required, individual counselling by the co-ordinator. Newpin will be extending the work it has done visiting mothers in nearby Guy's Hospital, both in the antenatal clinic and postnatal wards.

Anne Jenkins says, 'We are pretty hot on confidentiality.' Her records are open to individual mothers, but otherwise for her own use, and she would never contact another professional, say a GP, about the mother without her permission. The supporters, too, learn the importance of confidentiality, in order to maintain trust.

As well as home visiting and trips to Newpin, volunteers and the mothers they are helping may go out together, shopping or to a park. Some mothers have been particularly grateful for back-up in stressful situations such as going to the social security or housing office or to hospital. One of the purposes here is to help the supported mother to recognise her own competence in dealing with such agencies. The process of support may be two-way, with a referred mother helping her supporter through an unexpected bad patch.

In an evaluation of Newpin by psychologists Andrea Pound and Maggie Mills and psychiatrist Tony Cox, personal changes in the women referred were noted. A third of the previously depressed women recovered completely, and all but one of the rest became less depressed. Half of all the women in the study said their experiences in Newpin had helped them understand people better. Half, again, made friends for the first time at Newpin, and all but one said they had definitely confided in their volunteer or someone else there.

The most striking effects of involvement with Newpin are improved self-confidence and self-esteem – 'I learnt not to take the rubbish in,' says one mother. Improvements are also seen in relationships with partners, probably because the women learn to trust and confide in the Newpin setting and therefore begin to communicate more openly with their partners. Some men do come in to the centre informally, but Anne Jenkins would like to involve men more in the work of Newpin, possibly by setting up a men's group. One man, at least, felt he could be helpful to other men whose women are depressed.

One most heartening aspect of the scheme is its beneficial effects on the relationship between mothers and their children. Women feel ashamed and guilty when they hate or harm their children, usually too ashamed to seek help. Yet, at Newpin, 'the level of immediate physical chastisement of the children has reduced dramatically. More time is spent reasoning, playing with or consoling children . . . Mothers recognise other mothers' stress levels and will temporarily move in to take over a child when the infant becomes more demanding. This allows space for both mother and child to cool off. Normally, an insecure mother will see interventions as an indication she cannot cope, compounding her feelings of uselessness, but the trust already created seems to cancel out this fear.' Once mothers have developed self-respect, they can then respect their children and take responsibility for the burden of care. They also learn to accept themselves, that they cannot be good parents all the time.

Newpin can deal with PND by providing a supportive network around and after the birth. Women may be referred by, say, a health visitor who has defined PND as a crisis, but mothers do not see their situation as a crisis, says Anne Jenkins: 'They are simply up to the neck with daily problems.' She sees isolation, suspicion, and tunnel vision after the birth as factors leading to PND. 'It is easy for new mothers to slip into an isolation worse than that which society causes.' The slide into depression 'starts with self, but so many other things carry it on. Then authority takes over.' She feels that when women are hospitalised they take longer to recover. 'Even if they are raving when they go in, it would be better if they could stay out.' One mother with severe postnatal depression attended Newpin drop-ins daily because of the intensity of her suicidal feelings, but recovered.

Anne Jenkins, who was originally a midwife, feels increased hospitalisation of birth was a bad move and is very interested in the way birth affects women postnatally. She finds that mothers repress their birth experiences, or have had no opportunity to talk them out. This subject is brought up in training groups' self-awareness sessions and 'when the mothers are allowed to speak about their birth experiences they find it a terribly grieving time'. The birth experience is often felt to be 'a terrible violation'.

Of what particular value is a scheme like Newpin? 'The majority of people who come here are those very ones who are unable to motivate themselves to seek help before a crisis occurs, if indeed they are able to recognise they need help at all, yet are often in a state of apathy or confusion which can so often spiral downwards to require intensive professional intervention ... Involvement with Newpin seems to interrupt the spiral sufficiently to allow the individual to reassess their lives. Obviously this takes time but at relatively little cost, if it is weighed against the enormous expenses of using professional time and services.' Many of the mothers might have been considered unsuitable for conventional psychotherapy, yet Newpin, 'by providing a constantly available concerned person ("someone who is always there for you") and a safe base for the exploration of relationships, has been able to overcome the effects of early loss and disappointment in relationships which are too often considered irreversible.' (Pound et al) Both the giving and receiving of help outside a 'professional' setting seem to be sources of enhanced self-esteem, which can be actually undermined by the one-sidedness of professional help-giving.

Newpin uses the resources of goodwill and altruism in the community and, says Anne Jenkins, 'within its framework we can attempt to put back into the community what our society has been eroding, and that is belief in oneself and the human race. Our hope lies in the creation of a stable secure future generation.'

Chapter 6

What we can all do

Faced with a lack of general interest in the nature, origins and effects of PND, limited research, and conflicts of expert opinion, what can mothers do about emotional and mental disturbances that occur postnatally, for themselves and for each other, and how can their partners and families involve themselves? What mothers can do for themselves is dealt with in Chapter 7 and parts of Chapter 4; what others can do is considered here.

Partners, families and existing friends, because they know mothers before they even become pregnant, can do a lot to reduce the chances of PND occurring. They can make an effort to resolve long-standing ambivalencies or conflicts before a family is planned. They can be supportive and helpful during pregnancy and after the birth. Most partners and some relatives or friends will be able to encourage the mother through the birth. As postnatal depression is often easier to spot in someone else, they can keep an eye on new mothers, accept the responsibility of suggesting a mother needs help or at least to rethink what she is demanding of herself, or step in to protect a mother who meets unsympathetic medical response or is subjected to inappropriate or damaging treatment.

Mother and baby groups of all kinds have a helpful role to play. Those with which a mother is involved before the birth are strongly placed to stop PND before it starts, or at least contain it. If PND gets a hold, as depression is so crippling just because it attacks the will itself, and one problem in helping mothers with PND is overcoming their initial inertia in establishing new contacts and relationships, existing links are invaluable. Many mother and baby groups have informal connections with groups specifically concerned with helping mothers who have PND. These groups can defuse PND, reduce the time it lasts, or get sympathetic expert help. Other groups, set up to deal with specific problems relating to the birth, the baby, or parents' circumstances, offer general support plus practical advice based on firsthand experience. (For contact details, addresses of all types of groups and publications details, see Getting Help.)

INDIVIDUAL HELP

Because the early symptoms of depression are almost indistinguishable from extreme tiredness, which is expected in a new mother, postnatal depression (though not usually puerperal psychosis) frequently creeps up unnoticed and unnamed by partners, close family and friends. So being aware that PND exists and what its symptoms are is an important first step to being able to help (see over).

The simplest, and possibly the most effective, way to avert or cut short PND is to try to reduce all sources of stress for the mother. Good nutrition throughout pregnancy and from immediately after the birth strengthens the mother's resistance to unavoidable stress (see Chapter 4), as does getting as much rest as possible. Having a gentle birth is, of course, the best start to motherhood (see Chapter 2) and mothers may need help during pregnancy and in labour to achieve this. All those round a new mother can perform a valuable function by dissuading her from attempts to be superwoman (see Chapter 3) and offering practical help of all kinds. (It is no good telling a woman she should rest more without providing her with the opportunity to do so.) Those who are close can also give reassuring, confidence-building advice, that confirms the mother's instincts about her baby and how to look after it.

Nowadays many wives are in paid work and unable to offer their friends who are having babies the support they would like to give. The mothers of some new mothers may be working, too, and so unable to give their daughters very much help. But older family members, friends or neighbours, men as well as women, may be free to visit regularly or come and stay, and be glad to undertake a variety of tasks as well as being company.

Often relatives and close friends want to help mothers postnatally, whether they seem to be coping or have become disturbed, but are not sure of ways in which this can be done. Here are some suggestions for helping in practical ways, together with some advice on supporting mothers, which came out of a National Childbirth Trust study day on postnatal depression.

SIGNS TO WATCH OUT FOR

Symptoms of PND may be few or many, subtle or dramatic. No woman would undergo or show, all the following changes, but usually a variety of symptoms can be noticed. If a partner, relative or friend feels things are not quite right they should start by offering to lighten the mother's load in practical ways and by giving her opportunities to discuss how she feels. If she is adamant nothing is wrong when things are clearly getting worse then others who are close, or a member of a self-help group (see later) or a primary health care worker (see Chapter 5) should be enlisted to talk with the mother, allowing her to acknowledge her distress, then persuading her to accept help.

- extreme irritability
- tearfulness
- general anxiety
- panic
- tension
- manic energy
- unrealistic self-confidence
- brittle gaiety
- general disquiet
- despondency
- guilt
- feelings of incompetence and inadequacy
- inability to concentrate, remember or think clearly
- profound despair
- saying she wants to kill herself
- extreme fatigue
- general lethargy
- headaches
- general pains and feelings of being unwell
- insomnia
- early waking
- loss of appetite
- loss of sexual interest
- indifference to baby
- strange ideas about baby's needs
- neglect of baby
- morbid anxiety about baby
- violence towards baby
- saying baby would be better off dead

PRACTICAL ASSISTANCE

- have the baby, for periods as long as breastfeeding allows, or the mother does not mind being separated
- see she uses at least some of the time to rest and not to catch up on housework
- if she has other children, take them so that she can concentrate on the baby
- check she is eating properly
- invite her over for meals, or take dishes to her house, or offer to cook for her there
- offer to do specific household tasks, such as washing, ironing, mending or shopping
- go with her to self-help groups
- even if she has the use of a car offer her lifts
- babysit so she and her partner can go out without the baby

WAYS TO BE SUPPORTIVE

- encourage the mother to socialise and contact you at any time
- offer respect, shared experiences and acceptance; do not be smothering
- do not focus all your admiration on the baby
- avoid blaming her partner for problems or creating bad feeling between the couple
- listen to all she has to say
- do not argue: mental illness defies reason and logic so it is pointless to say, for example, that she should not feel afraid of going out
- do not let her feel guilty, nag or point out her shortcomings such as looking unkempt
- do not say things like 'pull yourself together' – that is precisely what she is unable to do
- utilise the expertise of other women who have been depressed, either individuals or group members
- if the mother is suicidal or expresses a desire to harm the baby, strongly suggest professional help
- if a suicidal mother is not admitted to hospital, make sure she is *never* left alone

Listening

Even if a mother appears to be fortunate in every way, well cared for and with a lovely, easy baby, emotional stress, rooted in the past or caused by her present relationships, may still take its toll. She may not understand what is wrong at all, or she may half know but be unable to communicate it. Either way, only listening will enable the problem to come out into the open where it can be dealt with.

Really listening is very hard and a Depressives Associated newsletter offers useful advice. 'The most important single factor in helping a troubled person is to listen: to pay attention with your eyes as well as your ears. Careful, sympathetic listening helps you to understand the problems better and has a healing effect on the one needing help. So, if someone asks you to listen – keep quiet, obtain the information, note the emotions, determine what is implied though not explicitly stated.' But, as the newsletter points out, 'It has been estimated that the average rate of thinking is about 400 words a minute. The average rate of speaking, however, has been estimated at about 120 words a minute. When someone is talking to you, what are you doing? More often than not, it is the human tendency for us to be thinking about what we are really going to say next. If this is so, are we really listening?'

Being told about a problem but not promptly seeing a solution may make the listener feel helpless and uncomfortable, so angry. Or it may dredge up disturbing and depressing emotions which the listener stills by cutting off the message. Truly listening is only possible if the hearer is prepared to take on board what is said and to consider change. If a partner, close relative or friend is afraid of this, they will block out what is being said, which is why comparative strangers who are not threatened by the implications of what they hear often make better listeners.

At some point, however, those close to a mother with PND will have to both open their ears and think about changes. In *Depression: The Way Out of Your Prison* Dorothy Rowe says, 'If someone close to you is depressed, and if you want that person to cease being depressed, then you have to be prepared to let that person change, and thus you yourself must change.' She considers that in listening we find out how a person sees a situation differently from us, and if there is any connection between the meaning that the person gives to

198

the situation and what she does. Explanations can become the starting points for change.

Partners

Little information is available to men on becoming fathers or dealing with PND. In west London the Ealing NCT Fathers Group made a contribution to putting this right by producing *Becoming a Father*. This booklet takes a very positive attitude, 'Becoming a father is not a chore, incidental to the "real world" of work, politics and the pub. Becoming a father can be the start of a whole new stage in your life,' while talking about the ambivalent and disturbing feelings that can result. Apprehension may alternate with enthusiasm, a man may find it hard to accept the pregnancy is real because it is not happening to him, seeing his partner as a mother may lead to confusions with his own mother, he may feel trapped and weighed down. For partners to be sensitive to each other's needs is the key. 'The problems start when either you or your partner assume that the other is feeling really confident and assured about the whole thing – this is not very likely, so it is important that you try to discuss both your hopes and your fears with each other and with other men or women who have gone through the same experiences.'

One way of trying to share the pregnancy would be to attend antenatal classes together. However, many hospital and clinic classes are for mothers only with one 'fathers' night' per course. This is often an inadequate and self-conscious exercise, with fathers feeling like outsiders and gaining very little. If more open classes are not available, reading good birth books together is likely to be more help (see Getting Help).

Tension and dissension are damaging emotions to bring to a birth, so exactly the kind of birth a woman hopes for, how far (or not) she is prepared to compromise, and what role her partner is to play should all be worked out beforehand. If a man's worries for the safety of his partner and their baby allow him to place too great a faith in routine technological interventions, and he tries to influence his partner against her instincts, he may undermine her confidence in herself and so her very ability to give birth freely. Women may remain deeply angry about a 'bad' birth for years afterwards. On the other hand, skilful support and encouragement may forge a new, deep and unbreakable bond between partners.

Not being aware of how you both feel and all the physical and emotional aspects of childbearing and parenthood lays the ground for misunderstanding and isolation, which can turn into depression in either partner. As the woman is usually under more intense and continuous stress, and as PND is generally regarded as an exclusively female manifestation, depression in the father is likely to be less immediately obvious and go undiagnosed. *Becoming a Father* points out, too, how depressingly empty the period straight after a birth can be for a new father. 'Men are not supposed to suffer from postnatal depression, but don't be suprised if you feel helpless, unable to cope, or even experience some quite strong negative feelings about life after birth and for the first few weeks of adjustment . . . It can help to talk things over with other men who have had, or are having, the same experiences.'

WHAT FATHERS CAN DO

An Association of Breastfeeding Mothers' leaflet offers some help to partners on what to expect and what to do. 'Life will never be quite the same after baby's arrival. Over the first few weeks the baby needs lots of his mother's attention. Support your wife with encouragement and practical help. Dads can cuddle and rock babies, talk to them, and help look after older children. Your help with the cooking, shopping and washing-up at this time is very valuable to your family. Protect your wife from too many visitors and from criticism from friends and relatives. It's a good idea to discuss together how you are going to look after the baby. You can help your wife realise that she doesn't have to compete with anyone else. Together you can work out priorities that make sense to you both. It can make a world of difference to your wife to know that you value what she is doing.'

Both partners can feel very fragile after a birth, and both may need support when the other one is unable to offer it. Becoming a father means growing up with a vengeance because, ideally, a man should be mature enough to set his own needs aside and give out to his wife who has to cope with the total dependency of a tiny baby. As circumstances are rarely ideal for anything, the next best thing is for a couple to recognise when they cannot meet each other's dependency needs at this time and be willing to turn to other people. If this is done openly, and both partners find support, the possible divisiveness of outside influences will be minimised. Some men undoubtedly find the constant presence of their mother-in-law, or a tight little group of their wife's female friends disconcerting, and feel resentful, excluded and undermined – partly because they may feel their relationship is absolutely private and should not be discussed, and partly because they may not know how or where to make friends for themselves.

Areas which can cause problems that go deeper than they appear are whether and when a mother returns to paid work, and breastfeeding. Breastfeeding mothers need a lot of support from their partners, because breastfeeding is best done in peace and quiet, free from worries, because it is very time and energy consuming, and because any adverse reactions or conflicting opinions can lead to feeding problems, which can in turn cause the mother a lot of emotional distress. *Becoming a Father* says that some men feel excluded by breastfeeding, wanting to help feed the baby themselves, and that 'It's a good idea to discuss infant feeding with your partner during pregnancy as some men find that they have rather ambivalent feelings about breastfeeding. How will you feel when "your" breasts are used almost exclusively by the baby? What about feeding in front of your friends – will you mind her exposing her breasts to them? Of course, it's not exactly a strip show, but breasts and sex have got rather confused in our present age.'

Feelings about mothers of new babies resuming paid work are much more complex than those relating to pure financial need. It is very important for a man to discover whether his partner really wants to return to her job quickly or feels she ought to or, alternatively, whether she longs to go straight back to her job but feels it would be wrong to leave the baby or fears her partner would think she was unwomanly and unnatural. And it is important for a man to know why he wants his partner to stay at home or work. Does her total dependency satisfy some need for ascendency or make him feel

201

more secure or more manly? Is her income really necessary, or does her working make her seem glamorous, more like his original girl-friend, and cut down the attention she gives to the baby?

Sex can be another minefield of hidden feelings. Whether they have PND or not, feel permanently exhausted or happy and lively, many women simply do not feel like resuming sexual relations soon after the birth (see Chapter 3). They may be absorbed in their baby, or be adjusting to their new persona, or have come to view their partner in a different light. Sometimes desire is one-sided on the part of the woman. Although his partner feels like making love, a man may develop inhibitions because of emotional responses to the birth, or because he somehow feels that becoming a mother has made his partner sexually unapproachable. *Becoming a Father* says, 'It is impossible to predict how you and your partner will feel about sex during pregnancy or after the baby is born,' and points out 'In many cultures a man is not expected to resume intercourse with his partner until the baby is weaned – anything from eighteen months to three years! Most men in this country don't expect to wait so long, but you should have no false expectations . . . Before the baby, your bodies were only for each other; now you have to share them with the baby. She will get physical satisfaction from nursing and cuddling the baby; so can you, but it may take time before the old flames of passion are rekindled.'

Whether existing dissatisfaction with a marriage can cause depression postnatally, or PND breaks up marriages is a chicken and egg situation, but undeniably living with a woman who is depressed is a strain. The atmosphere becomes poisoned with repressed anger, lack of trust, and insecurity. Dorothy Rowe says that depressed people give out ambivalent messages – 'Help me/stay away' – and this is painful and confusing for their partner. But, however hard it is, listening is vital. 'Understanding means seeing connections,' and that is not possible without seeing how your partner views the situation. PND cannot be separated from a relationship because 'depression is not some *thing* inside a person but it is the way that person relates to her-self and the people around her. A spouse is just as much involved in the depression as the person who is depressed.' Some men want to view their partner's depression separately and not in the context of their relationship, perhaps because they fear their own depression or their underlying anger will be revealed.

Some couples get nowhere in looking at their relationship because they fail to realise that one or other or both of them are re-living their parents' marriages. Or the man may not admit (or realise) that his wife has become depressed because she is utterly drained by the burden of sustaining a dependent infant and an emotionally dependent partner.

A man may be blind to the fact that he limits what his partner undertakes, ostensibly out of protective love – 'I don't want you overdoing things' – but actually to keep her available to supply his needs, practical and emotional, or keeps her at home so that he will not lose her. He may actually have got her pregnant to keep her to himself; she may sense this and feel trapped and bitter. If the marriage is an unacknowledged power struggle, depression in the woman after birth may be a subconscious way of righting the balance at a time when she feels particularly powerless.

Dorothy Rowe has some good advice on dealing with a partner's depression. 'Listen and share. Listening means accepting the other person's pain . . . Don't push it away [or run away from it] by belittling it or denying that it exists. Accept the pain, stay with it, and offer, not advice, but a comforting hand or a shoulder to cry on.'

PND support groups

To prevent and deal with PND it is vital for mothers to have sufficient contact with adults in the postnatal period. This will provide sympathy, warmth, mental stimulus, practical help and advice. NCT mother Olive Farrow says, 'Depression has taught me many good things, and one of these is this – that our mind needs stimulus, and if it gets nothing at all to occupy itself with, then it will ponder on the sad and unhappy things of past and present. We need people so much. Going out and making friends can be a difficult task at first, but we are rewarded for our good efforts.'

Television presenter Esther Rantzen says she came across no mention of PND when she was preparing to have her first baby. After the birth she found herself victim to uncontrollable bursts of weeping, and still she did not realise what was wrong with her. Her salvation came through talking to other mothers, not all of whom had suffered from PND, but who were all able to listen, and who showed they were not bored. She was also reassured by those friends who had suffered from PND, when they convinced her that she was neither a freak, nor insane, and by the very fact that they had recovered.

Isolation is the biggest creator of depression, and the biggest barrier to discovery and recovery. In a *Mother and Baby* survey, says writer Vivienne Stocks, 'over half the mothers complaining of depression received no help and muddled through on their own.' While, 'One of the surprising facts unearthed by Cambridge researchers was that only two of the depressed women in their study had sought help from their GPs, and though some had discussed their problems with a partner, friend or relative, most had simply suffered in silence.'

Even if a mother had a close network of family and friends, unless they, too, have babies and toddlers, it is often easier to see other mothers who had previously been strangers, but who share the same timetables, needs, problems and recent birth experience. This is why joining any group for housewives and mothers is good, but postnatal support groups provide particularly relevant contact. For mothers who already have PND, specific postnatal depression support groups are run by ex-sufferers.

Self-help groups, run by people whose primary qualification for supporting mothers is that they are mothers, too, in dealing with PND are often seen as second-best to professional aid – appealing to only one class of woman, limited in usefulness to mild cases of PND, a back-up for correct medical treatment, or a last resort for mothers who 'fail' to respond to conventional help. Sometimes groups are condemned outright as a load of meddling amateurs.

But psychiatrist Dr Desmond Bardon, adviser to the NCT, says that groups have a very valuable role to play in PND. 'Depression and its treatment is a highly complicated subject and the pooled opinion of a number of experienced women who can offer love and all sorts of support to a depressed mother may be much safer for her than the fashionable or deep-seated prejudices of either a well-meaning or hostile professional,' he says in the NCT booklet on PND.

Friendship is what most mothers seek and find in support groups. Friendship is born at the moment one person says to another, 'You too? I thought I was the only one!' says a Depressives Associated newsletter. And, very importantly, group settings are in themselves therapeutic – the whole is greater than the sum of the parts. In self-help groups, as in group psychotherapy, becoming part of a group can be, in itself, sufficient to effect change and so improvement in mood and optimism.

According to the late Leonard D Borman, founder of the Self-Help Center, an American nation-wide research and information clearing house based in Illinois, 'Groups are finding new ways of understanding and helping the professionals understand. They offer a tremendous amount of hope for people ready to throw in the towel.' He dismissed the notion that because groups are not professional they may offer wrong information or lead people astray as 'hogwash, not true'. Borman said studies showed a growing number of people were finding support groups a valuable aid in learning to cope with problems, and that members have better mental health than non-members with comparable problems. He felt that one reason for the growth in self-help groups was 'increasingly people are taking more control of their lives. They want to become more informed and more involved in making decisions which affect them.' He said that some of the mechanisms identified by research as making groups effective were an immediate sense of identity, the healing power of helping others, the exchange of information, and instant support on the telephone.

Psychologist Denis O'Connor feels that caring can only be done by someone who has troubles of their own, and quotes the founder of analytical psychology Carl Jung – 'only the injured physician can heal'. He believes touching is an important way to show caring and create a bond – cuddling or holding hands. This is likely to happen in a more spontaneous way within a group of mothers than between a professional and client.

Women friends and acquaintances may suggest to a lonely or distressed mother that she joins a group they know, health professionals may recommend groups, or mothers may approach groups themselves. Self-help groups vary in the sort of women who belong to them, the way they are run, the degree of severity of PND they can cope with, their beliefs on causes and treatments, and whether or not they have close links with outside professionals. The work of some very different well-established organisations is described next, after some suggestions on how group volunteers can help mothers.

HOW TO HELP

When faced with a mother who is depressed postnatally we often feel inadequate and do not know what we can do. The Pacific Post Partum Support Society in Vancouver compiled this list of what mothers said volunteers had done that helped them when they had PND.

- listened
- sounded as if she cared
- gave of herself
- gave a feeling of being in touch when I cut myself off
- was honest with you
- wasn't shocked, she was understanding
- was on your side
- gave praise and support for every effort made
- wasn't judgemental
- brought things into perspective
- knew
- was an example of an all-right person who came through a dreary time
- the fact that she had made it was inspiring and encouraging to me
- helped recognise small successes and efforts when they weren't terribly apparent
- helped keep you on a feeling level
- wasn't ashamed of what happened to her
- told me that I mattered
- was willing to give you the time
- told me that she enjoyed talking with me
- was there when I really needed her
- helped me see 'selfish' as a different thing
- nothing was too small
- her openness made a trust
- wasn't embarrassed by her own faults, flaws, problems
- helped me see that I could stand on my own
- made me feel very warm
- made me feel comfortable and relaxed
- reiterated 'It gets better'
- was someone to talk to
- was a safety valve
- enjoyed hearing the good things as well as the bad
- gave me the feeling that I didn't have to be alone
- could laugh at herself and had a good sense of humour
- accepted my feelings – no matter what they were
- allowed me to be her friend
- helped me work out my feelings
- helped me get in touch with my feelings

- booted me when I needed it
- gave me encouragement
- could tell if I had feelings other than what I was saying
- I learned that she was a person and not a god – and that helped me
- I knew she had many problems of her own
- the difficulties she had with her child were really similar to the ones I was having
- asked questions that I needed to be asked
- was there
- told me when she couldn't be there
- made me appreciate that there were positive things happening – not just negative
- showed confidence in me
- gave many suggestions on how to handle certain situations
- asked me how I felt and accepted how I felt
- shared her feelings with me
- offered enough alternatives that one was bound to work
- showed me that she was still improving which gave me courage to face downs
- it was OK to have a down day
- in talking to me, if she found something that would help she would appreciate me for it

The Association for Post-Natal Illness

This group stresses its professional links. 'The Association is run by a Committee which contains a Professor of Chemical Pathology, a Consultant Psychiatrist, a Consultant Obstetrician, a General Practitioner and a Biochemist. There is also a Scientific Advisory Committee which contains five Consultant Psychiatrists, two Consultant Obstetricians and a Pharmacologist.' It has four areas of activity – education, information, support and research.

The association first reaches mothers through a leaflet 'which describes the baby blues and postnatal depression' and is available free from health authorities, maternity units and antenatal instructors. 'The leaflet seeks to make women more aware of the illness without alarming them. It is hoped that women who read the leaflet and subsequently develop the illness will seek medical care earlier.'

Once mothers have read a leaflet (picked up somewhere like a clinic or sent on application by post to the association) and decide they want help, then they receive further information. If they apply for support, a volunteer will contact the mother by telephone. Volunteers are mothers who have completely recovered from PND. 'Depressed mothers are phoned at regular intervals throughout their illness and the recovery period. Most mothers find it an enormous relief to talk to someone who really understands how they feel.'

Founder Clare Delpech emphasises the need for early and better recognition of PND, by the mother, those around her or professionals. 'The cases we see are just the tip of the iceberg,' she says. 'People need to be more aware of the very real possibility of postnatal depression; too many just suffer alone.'

When volunteer supporters phone mothers they try to get them to express what is wrong with them, perhaps by comparing their feelings with those described in the leaflet. They may be tired, lonely or clinically depressed. Women will say they have been feeling 'so poorly', but not that they have PND. If the replies indicate to the volunteer that the mother is unwell, they will very firmly suggest that the mother sees a doctor.

Clare Delpech believes in referring to professionals because she worries about seriously ill women being harmed. 'I would rather not start to help than cause harm. Some self-help groups are well-meaning but could cause great harm in ignorance.' What she feels her association can do is firstly increase awareness – 'The more people know, the quicker they become aware of what is happening.' Then 'offering hope is vital, whoever we are dealing with. Our role is to encourage them to do something for themselves . . . Women who are seriously ill become hopeless. It is a drowning syndrome . . . Sometimes their friends don't even get in the door so they don't know what is happening and can't help . . . It is alarming how many women say they counted out the tablets until they had an overdose – they have been on the brink.'

Clare Delpech does not believe that PND can be completely avoided, but taking certain steps may reduce its severity, especially after a subsequent birth. Fatigue plays a big role and rest is very important. 'Vulnerable' mothers would be wise to plan a lot of support, plan to be useless for several weeks. If they have no family, support is worth going without something else to pay for.

She estimates that a third of women who contact the association can be helped by progesterone treatment (see Chapter 4). When Clare Delpech had PND herself, as a biochemist she became interested in possible hormonal influences on the illness. She is now convinced that PND can be at least affected by hormonal changes, if not actually caused by it. She feels that where there has been no psychiatric history prior to postnatal depression or puerperal psychosis, then it is probably due to biochemical causes. She has become convinced of this because 'the vast majority of women I meet are so down to earth, so keen to get better. They are enormously well-adjusted, have no life crises, yet postnatal depression hits them badly.'

The association keeps a close watch on research into PND all round the world through its scientific secretary Ellen Goudsmit, and Clare Delpech finds it upsetting that comparatively little research is done and that no new treatments are being offered. 'Nothing useful has emerged in the past five or six years. It's just the same old antidepressants.'

National Childbirth Trust

This organisation, whose work started in 1956 with a group of mothers, now has some 10,000 full members, 320 branches and groups, and is internationally recognised. The NCT aim 'to help families achieve greater enjoyment in childbirth and parenthood. Antenatal classes, support with breastfeeding, and practical help, support and contact after the baby is born are the most important aspects of our work.' They spread information and give support through publishing leaflets, booklets and books and arranging study days, but primarily by friendly personal contact.

The general postnatal support network 'consists of women giving each other whatever they, as unique individuals, are able to,' says NCT member Maureen Thomas. 'We do not provide answers – there aren't always answers to give – but we do offer friendship. We are probably the only organisation which does this – supporting people because they have babies, not because they have problems. This is not, and cannot be, counselling – because it is an informal, mutually beneficial, relationship between equal individuals. Its very simplicity is such that its value can be understated.'

Depressed or disturbed mothers are included in the postnatal support network but, because many have a great need to talk to someone who has had PND and recovered, some branches have postnatal supporters with a special interest in the subject, arising from their personal experiences. Sometimes branches have links with specific PND support groups. In the NCT booklet *Mothers Talking About Postnatal Depression* the work of a PND support group in Bristol is described. Their aim is 'to act on a purely mother-to-mother, non-professional basis in order to provide one-to-one support and friendship and a mutual support group for husbands and wives who are experiencing and/or have recovered from a postnatal illness.' The supporters have experienced some form of postnatal illness themselves, and have been recovered for at least a year. They are themselves well supported, because the work is emotionally demanding. The group has a medical adviser who can be consulted as necessary.

The way in which NCT branches and the groups with which they have links provide help for mothers with PND varies in organisation and style, according to what members prefer, but all offer friendly, caring, non-advisory support. Supporters, those being supported, and perhaps other mothers, may go to meetings and coffee mornings, as and when they feel like it, visit other members, or merely receive the occasional newsletter. Sometimes mothers want only phone calls and no other contact; sometimes they do not want individual support.

In the Aylesbury district the hospital obstetric liaison service which deals with PND and is run by Dr Diana Riley (see Chapter 5) has maintained close links with the local NCT from the beginning. 'Discussion groups with members in each local branch have resulted in better awareness of early symptoms and better postnatal support for members. In High Wycombe, NCT teachers have been involved with regular group therapy meetings held at the hospital. These groups originally provided a link with the hospital for recently discharged patients, but later widened their scope to include outpatients as well. A similiar group has recently been set up by NCT postnatal supporters in Amersham, and has produced a useful leaflet for its members.'

The Blackpool and Fylde NCT branch have co-operated with their local Community Health Council and health professionals to produce a short, straightforward leaflet, *After Baby What Next?* This covers the emotional after-effects of childbirth, alerts mothers to the possibility of PND, and suggests ways of coping, who to contact for help and some useful publications. Liz Evans of the branch says, 'We have found the booklet useful, and the links forged during its drafting between ourselves, the health and social services professionals have been invaluable both to us and mums with PND. We all trust each other's opinions and place in helping PND sufferers much more.'

NCT members are aware that fathers need support, too – in their own right and because the well-being of the father is crucial to the well-being of mother and baby. Fathers are welcome at antenatal classes and Liz Waumsley (former chair of the national postnatal committee) says in *New Generation*, 'For many expectant fathers it is the point at which they really begin to feel involved in the pregnancy – as they realise that many of their feelings are shared by the other men, as they listen to those who are already fathers talking about their experiences, and as they become more informed. Many expectant parents seem to find that a discussion on "what we think it will be like after the birth" enables them to put into words feelings and worries that they had not expressed even to each other.' After the birth fathers occasionally work with each other in separate groups, but are mainly helped by supporters thinking of the needs of the family as a whole and, perhaps, directing a mother's attention to how fathers often need to feel more involved or how they might find added responsibility a strain.

The need for partners to be supported, too, is referred to again in the NCT PND booklet, this time in talking about severe depression. 'It is important to accept that you cannot always help, except by being available as and when needed. During her recovery period, which may be lengthy and "up and down", a woman who could not previously take advantage of what was offered may be glad to do so. Her self-confidence is likely to need rebuilding, and a loving, uncritical acceptance combined with encouragement will help a great deal. Her partner, too, is likely to feel shattered by the experience.'

Regardless of whether or not they have PND, some mothers have particular requirements in postnatal support. For instance, more and more women are returning to paid work while their babies are still infants, some very soon after the birth, and they are frequently at their most vulnerable when looking for someone to care for their child. They have particular stresses and conflicts to deal with and need someone to discuss their new problems and experiences with. In response many NCT branches have established working mothers' groups, or have a postnatal supporter who can provide specific advice.

Sue Smith, NCT member and Clapham Working Mothers Group founder, says that there is a growing body of mothers who have to cope with the triple responsibilities of a job, motherhood and employing someone to care for their baby or children. She felt a special group was needed because, 'On returning to work I felt very isolated; I did not know anyone else with a small baby, working or not, and having a full-time job I was excluded from participating in the normal NCT postnatal support network of weekday functions.'

In May 1984 the known working mothers' groups decided to form a national organisation to act as an umbrella for local groups and the Working Mothers Association was launched in January 1986. It operates independently and some NCT working mothers are members of both organisations. The WMA produce their own publications, including *The Working Mother's Handbook*.

Mothers who are disabled in various ways also have certain special requirements. The NCT believe that their support system of mother-to-mother contact has the potential to provide a vital source of help and reassurance. They followed up the publication of their booklet *The Emotions and Experiences of Some Disabled Mothers* with a study day. What came out of this is that the main problem facing disabled parents is lack of advice and information, and that disabled parents need to be in control of the situation. Even if they cannot do certain things physically they must make the decisions as to what happens and when. As well as receiving support within the NCT, mothers with disabilities can receive information and support of various kinds that enables them to stay in charge from a growing number of self-help groups.

With regard to PND, the great advantage for mothers of belonging to the NCT is that, because mothers are likely to have joined during pregnancy or soon after the birth, they are already known to other members who can explain that PND exists and what the symptoms are, and spot it in mothers who have not realised what is wrong with them. Hopefully, being part of a network and already having reliable friends may prevent some cases of PND happening at all and reduce the severity of or cut short others. If a mother has become deeply depressed without anyone realising it, the specific expertise of PND supporters can ensure she gets appropriate professional help swiftly and see her through the worst times.

Sheffield Post-Natal Depression Support Group

Two mothers who had been very disturbed after the births of their children decided to form a local group to help other mothers, using their own experiences. Agnes Burns attributes her depression to a complex of reasons, explained to her by Depressives Associated who she contacted. All her family lived abroad, she had lost her friends when she came to this country and through moving twice when she was pregnant, had no energy for any interests, at first she, her husband and baby Jamie were short of money and lived in one room and, perhaps, there was a hormonal imbalance after the birth (see Chapter 4).

PND hit her suddenly in the form of terrible panic. She felt utterly exhausted and feared she would hurt her baby, especially when he cried. This idea shocked her and made her feel she was going mad. Agnes then became suicidal. Her GP gave her antidepressants, which helped. But beginning to understand what PND is and to accept that she had it eased her tension, lessened the panic and helped recovery. 'Slowly I began to meet other mums and became involved in our local playgroup, so I learned that other mothers had gone through exactly the same experience, which gave a tremendous feeling of relief.'

Carol Philpotts developed puerperal psychosis after the birth of Adam. 'I rejected the baby, I could not recall the labour or birth and was unable to cope with breastfeeding.' Hospital staff were unsympathetic, advice was conflicting. She became manic, was admitted to the mother and baby unit of a psychiatric hospital, where she suffered hallucinations and delusions. She was treated with major tranquillisers and antidepressants, plus ECT. 'The ECT was a horrifying experience, but did succeed in ridding me of my delusions and hallucinations. I was left dopey, sleepy, wracked with self-doubt; totally without self-confidence.'

After leaving psychiatric hospital it took her a whole year to get back to normal. Carol feels she was poorly prepared for what happened. 'I was not warned about postnatal depression and I was ignorant of possible puerperal psychosis. I did not know the realities of motherhood – how much *hard* work it all is and also what a full-time responsibility a small baby is.' She believes that her

213

depression was largely due to hormonal factors, and if she had another baby would ask for preventative hormone treatment.

The Sheffield group help other mothers by presenting a realistic picture of motherhood – 'The picture of motherhood is often a false one; glowing mother and rosy child is often not the reality,' and by providing friendship – 'Do not stay lonely, isolated and frightened with your baby. Come and join our informal self-help group. We offer reassurance, support and information in a relaxed friendly atmosphere. You do not have to be afraid of sharing your fears with us.' They also give details of how to get hormone treatment and maintain close links with other organisations that can offer support, practical advice or help – general or especially relating to children.

In their group leaflet they say that one of the reasons for PND 'is a severe reaction towards a situation of which we had no previous experience.' They stress the tremendous adjustments a new mother has to make and the many losses birth entails, plus the isolation it brings and the deep fears that can result. 'The only way to overcome these fears is by talking to other mothers who have been through the same thing and who have recovered. In this way self-confidence can slowly be restored. Because of the conventional treatment of depression – pills, hospital, electric shock treatment – many mothers never come to understand the *reason* for their condition and stay ill for a very long time.

'We must learn to accept that love towards our new baby does not always come naturally. New mums often suffer from guilt because they lack warm feelings towards their baby.'

Agnes received preventative hormone treatment for her second birth and did not become ill again. She says, 'Here in Sheffield it is very difficult to get natural progesterone treatment. Psychiatrists oppose the treatment and keep telling us how wonderful ECT plus drugs are. I find this a very cruel treatment. The mother comes home, drugged up, and still full of anxiety and unable to cope, and she has severe memory loss. Once you come out of psychiatric hospital, there is no help or follow-up for mothers. Terrible! After three months in hospital it is a terrible shock, to be *alone* again.

'Well, if these psychiatrists could hear the mother afterwards, they might get a better idea of the whole situation. Mothers complain bitterly – they say: "I never want to go through that again." Also, there is no *prevention* with all this ECT and heavy drug treatment and that worries mothers who want another baby. The second time mothers are offered antidepressants while they are pregnant. Many refuse, for fear of harming the baby. Well, I am sure there are many other reasons for PND besides hormone trouble, but I wish they would give this safer and gentler treatment a fair trial.'

Agnes had a home confinement for her second birth and feels that this made PND less likely. She also says, 'Psychiatrists want to keep dealing with the brain, only with the mal-function. They don't want to think, or admit, that PND could also have social plus physical causes. If they admitted that, then they would have to start changing. They would be obliged to *listen* to the depressed mum – a thing they rarely want to do (too time-consuming).

'I can only see change if midwives, health visitors plus mothers are going to push for change. It will take time. With depression generally people complain of doctors not wanting to listen plus no sympathy. All surgeries should have a few good counsellors attached. It all boils down to giving the depressed person some *time*.'

Depressives Associated

The main aim of this charity is to encourage people to befriend each other, individually, in their groups or in the other groups they work with. DA was the outcome of mothers' responses to the television play *Baby Blues*. The author, Nemone Lethbridge, had been a victim of PND, and her play on its problems elicited 1500 letters from mothers. Midwife Janet Stevenson, who had suffered from PND herself, undertook to respond to the letters, then founded Depressives Associated to help women whose problem was being ignored. Now the association hopes to encourage mothers who get PND to seek help much earlier.

DA set out to encourage those in a negative state of mind to learn how to be positive again, mainly by 'sharing in caring'. Mrs Stevenson feels that 'those suffering from depression, or a mind-reversal state, are so emotionally isolated, and feel so alienated from life that they, themselves, being so troubled, are longing for loving understanding.' DA also think that doctors do not really understand depression and that they treat the symptoms rather than the causes. 'For a thousand depressives, there will be a thousand causes. We try to work in small groups where the knowledge of one depressive person can be used to help another.'

Mrs Stevenson says, 'One thing I have found out about PND is that many husbands cannot take the hassle of fatherhood.' They escape, leaving the mother trapped with a crying baby. She is concerned that unrecognised PND has an ongoing effect on the whole family. 'Violence and child sexual abuse often ties in with PND. When a husband cannot understand what is happening to his wife, he may abuse her or the child.' The children may be affected even further as the family disturbance perpetuates itself. If the couple divorce and the wife remarries, 'Many step-parents find that children will not accept them. These men only know one way to show their superiority, not by beatings which would upset their wives, but by forcing sexual acts, and hoping the young person won't tell anyone.' The deep-buried wound of incest stays with the victim until her own marriage, pregnancy and childbirth reactivate it and she, in turn, becomes disturbed postnatally.

In conjunction with the Sheffield PND Support Group, DA have produced a booklet on PND *You Are Not Alone* which explains what has happened and how others can help, and emphasises recovery. DA, as well as support, offer counselling plus advice on adequate nutrition and how to breathe properly and relax, 'With the stresses of modern life, it is very hard to keeep well,' says Shirley Toms, a primary school teacher specialising in movement and dance who set up the London branch of DA. She has also established SAD (Society Against Depression), a mental health information service for Londoners which will reach women with PND, amongst others.

If a mother has PND Shirley Toms thinks her immediate need is for other women with small babies who know how difficult it is being a mother. As well as emotional support mothers can offer practical help, like taking the baby for an hour, and practical advice from their own experience. Unless a mother with PND is severely disturbed, Shirley would say to her, 'Yes, it is damned hard, but you can and will get through it,' then see she has continual support and encouragement. She feels that mothers who are deeply disturbed very often need a good rest, and points out that extreme tiredness can even cause hallucinations.

Rest is difficult to get because new mothers are mentally and socially isolated in their responsibility for the baby, partly because 'We are anti-child in British society.' PND is often ignored – 'Many sufferers are dismissed as neurotic or hysterical or having "women's little troubles".' Where treatment is given Shirley feels, 'We have to be wary that it is not just telling women or providing the means for them to adjust to their lot rather than improving the conditions that caused their distress in the first place.'

Shirley believes that one of the reasons women become depressed is that we are such a hypocritical and repressed society. ' "Thou shalt appear to be happy" is a maxim of Western thinking, and to show one's emotions is taboo. Touch is not part of our puritan society.' But keeping a stiff upper lip keeps emotions bubbling below the surface, to erupt at some later date. She wonders if this is why there is so much wife and baby battering. In women, where emotion often cannot be expressed as anger, the anger turns inwards to become self-hatred, guilt and depression. Or the trapped emotions and feelings of powerlessness can lead to a state of learned helplessness. When this attitude conflicts with the demands of motherhood, depression can result.

Shirley says, 'Most people don't want to face their pain,' so, in working to help them, she has to get them to talk out their loss and pain, and also make sense of it. 'It isn't enough simply to let people off-load onto you.' Talking with someone sympathetic enough for a mother to feel safe in opening up, yet strong enough to encourage her to look at how things really are, can start a healing process that results in a gradual return of trust, hope and joy. As Shirley Toms says, 'Most people have lost the child inside themselves.'

Pacific Post Partum Support Society

This unique service started in response to a request from women in the Vancouver community who had become depressed after the birth or adoption of a child. 'These women said they had been helped most by other women who had been through the experience and offered to talk to women referred to them by the local crisis centre,' says Joann Robertson, one of the founders of Canada's Vancouver Postpartum Counselling Program which has become the Post Partum Support Society (see Getting Help). The original programme consisted of limited one-way telephone contact, about once a week. It expanded with the services of two students, one taking a master's degree in social work and one in nursing.

'The students had limited theoretical and experiential backgrounds in this area and were not able to get much useful information from the medical and psychiatric literature.' They found lack of agreement and widespread confusion in the use of the labels blues, postnatal depression and puerperal psychosis. Nor was the literature helpful in regard to treatment as it was based on admissions to psychiatric hospitals and mainly concerned the use of drugs and ECT. 'It became obvious that the people who had the most knowledge about postpartum depression were women who had experienced it.' Through a newspaper article women with PND or those who had got over it were asked to contact the programme. From that, a group of women was formed who supported each other through daily telephone contact and through weekly meetings led by the students.

The society developed by learning – first from women how they feel and behave when depressed, and second what helps them to recover. They have a handful of social workers as staff and a large number of volunteer supporters, all of whom were helped by the society at some time. The staff do a lot of liaising within the programme and with various professional and community groups about PND and related issues such as child abuse and the effects of depression on the family. They also offer family counselling, and individual counselling of both mothers and fathers. Fathers are welcomed to their own regular information meetings.

Through dealing with well over 1000 mothers they have discovered who in their catchment area tends to get PND. 'She is 27 years old, married, middle-class and has two years of post-secondary education. The pregnancy is planned, both parents attend prenatal classes; the father is present for the delivery. The mother chooses to breastfeed. We have not found a significant incidence of previous depression in these women, nor have we found many to be immature or having poor coping mechanisms prior to their postpartum depression. Some have themselves experienced inadequate parenting, but many have not.' Women who do not fit this profile also get PND, but 'It is useful to note that the woman who is at risk is often the very one who is expected to make a trouble-free transition into motherhood.'

In the programme the volunteer has an essential role. 'What helps women to recover is being able to talk to someone who really understands how they are feeling and what it is like to be at home with small children. The volunteer spends time identifying with the woman, reassuring her that she is not unique, that she is not going crazy, that how she feels is shared by other women. She assists the woman in setting realistic goals for herself so that she can begin to assume control over her life and regain her sense of self.'

In the way the society works, 'women are participants in their therapy in a much different way than is allowed for in traditional therapy. When the helper is perceived as having all the knowledge (and therefore the power) women are kept in a dependent role.' They believe that the sharing of information between women 'helps to break down the role boundaries between the helper and the helped which can keep women from recognising their own knowledge and strength.'

SPECIAL NEEDS

There is an enormous range of organisations and groups, national and local, that aim to provide women with a social life, domestic and childbearing information, and aid when they are in difficulties. Some, such as the National Women's Register, deliberately emphasise interests outside the home. Organisations like the Women's Institutes and Townwomens Guilds have very broad interests and are influential in bringing certain aspects of women's problems to government notice. There are many mother and toddler groups, from small informal gatherings to national networks like Mama (Meet-a-Mum Association) and the Pre-School Playgroups Association. Some organisations, like the National Council for One Parent Families, are for sections of the community with particular needs. All these groups offer help, support and a forum for the exchange of information, but those most likely to reach mothers with PND are the breastfeeding networks and the crisis groups helping with specific problems that parents have with their babies.

Breastfeeding

Tiredness and depression in the mother, crying and wakefulness in the baby and difficulties in breastfeeding are linked as cause and effect in many ways. Lack of sleep and inadequate nutrition can lead to poor milk supply which produces a miserable fractious baby. Crying and wakefulness with various causes (see later) can physically exhaust the mother and make her feel inadequate. Apparent inability to breastfeed can leave a mother feeling disappointed and a failure. And the timing and pace of stopping breastfeeding affects hormonal levels (see Chapter 4).

One NCT mother described to her breastfeeding counsellor how down she became after the birth of her son. 'I couldn't be bothered with anything. I was so tired, so desperately tired – yet I couldn't sleep. Soon I couldn't cope. The two most predominant feelings were of extreme loneliness and complete inadequacy.' Then she had to give up breastfeeding. 'I was totally unprepared for the aggressive way I felt towards my baby when I fed him by bottle. I wanted the job over and done with in seconds. I felt angry because he wouldn't hurry up and was offended at his obvious enjoyment of his feeds. I felt as though he had rejected me and I, in turn, was beginning to reject him. These thoughts left me badly shaken and very frightened . . . I could see it was illogical to feel guilty and inadequate about my failure to breastfeed, nevertheless that was how I felt.'

Breastfeeding is obviously the way mothers were designed to nourish and comfort their newborns and, after being frowned on by the experts, is now medically back in fashion, its nutritional, health protection and emotional values having been 'scientifically' proven. Yet many mothers find it difficult. The Thomas Coram Research Unit in one study found feeding was the most common problem during the hospital stay after birth and continued to be so (for up to a year) for one-third of mothers. One reason for problems could be the double messages women receive about their physical functions, including breastfeeding – it is a praiseworthy way to feed a baby, but must be done furtively. Other reasons are lack of information, rigid notions (usually on the part of professionals), conflicts of opinion, and not receiving enough practical help to be able to get the requisite peace and quiet to feed.

Women in more traditional countries breastfeed successfuly even when they are low-weight, have multiple births or have to resume hard work very soon. A true commitment to breastfeeding by professionals in hospitals, better training, and the use of lactation nurses could do a lot to help mothers establish breastfeeding. In a Cardiff study, the group supported by a lactation nurse who offered consistent advice and encouragement had significantly more mothers breastfeeding at four weeks and at each check up to six months.

The effectiveness of support is no news to groups like the La Leche League and the Association of Breastfeeding Mothers who offer information, encouragement and support from mothers who have breast-fed their babies to others who wish to do so. And the groups are well aware of the harmful effects 'failure' to breastfeed has on mothers who want to nurture their infants in that way. Peggy Thomas, general secretary of the ABM, says, 'If a mother wants to breastfeed and doesn't, she is laying herself open to problems, depression being one of them.'

Through leaflets, talks, group meetings and individual contact the self-help groups provide detailed advice on breastfeeding that is not available elsewhere. In a society where many women have little or no experience of living with a baby they stress the importance of having realistic expectations. The groups are very flexible in their approach, believing that mothers must trust their instincts about how often to feed their babies (perhaps every two hours), for how long (maybe 45 minutes a feed) and until what age (when the child wants to stop, even if it is a toddler on solids). They offer reassuring, confidence-building advice – 'It's not really anybody else's business how or where you feed your baby. Do it your way.' (ABM leaflet)

In spite of being dedicated to the virtues of breastfeeding, group counsellors and leaders are sensitive to the fact that some mothers find it a terrible tie or actually a distressing or depressing experience, and agree that it is then better to admit these feelings and stop. Mothers who have PND or have sleep problems, despite strong feelings for wanting to continue breastfeeding, may find that giving it up takes an enormous weight off their minds, sometimes because the responsibility for feeding is then shared with their partner.

One of the most important functions of the breastfeeding groups in a hard, brisk, emotionally repressed society is to give mothers 'permission' to enjoy their babies – to allow their softer feelings full play, through attentive observation of the baby to be able to read its messages of need and love, and to learn to let themselves respond to them (see Chapter 7).

Wakefulness

'I didn't realise how alert and active she would be . . . I thought at this stage it would be all feed and sleep. It has all been a bit of a shock.' Thus the mother of a three-month-old baby sums up the dismay felt by parents at the discrepancy between their expectation that a small baby will sleep for long periods of time and the reality of an infant who scarcely seems to close its eyes. So called sleeping problems are frequent, affecting at least an estimated one-third of parents, and cover babies not sleeping many hours out of the 24, not sleeping much in the day, not wanting to go to sleep at night, frequent night waking or waking for extended periods at night. These babies do not suffer from insufficient sleep, but their parents do. Lack of preparedness can be as bad as the actual lack of rest. Because mothers are not adequately warned of the time and effort caring for a wakeful newborn involves, they may expect to fit everything in as usual and become frustrated, exhausted and depressed when they cannot.

Insufficient sleep at night and, worse, interrupted sleep cycles, can quickly turn anyone into a wreck. Everything becomes too much, the desire for sleep becomes an obsession, and the slide into clinical depression is easy. Being woken constantly soon assumes the form of torture, with dread compounding the reality. If that is not bad enough mothers are usually made to feel responsible for preventing the baby waking their partner 'because he works all day' (caring for a baby and running a home full-time do not qualify as 'real' work). Then, all too often, mothers are blamed for the problem – they must be doing something wrong.

Talking to other mothers with the same problem may or may not provide clues to what is causing the wakefulness, but it certainly eases the guilt, sense of failure and isolation. The National Association of Parents of Sleepless Children was started by the parents of two wakeful children who were 'dismayed by the lack of sympathy, understanding and reasonable advice offered.' Their main aim has been 'to help assuage the guilt parents are made to feel when their children don't sleep as much as they are supposed to.' Their second aim has been to re-educate parents, health visitors and doctors into accepting that 'all children are different and that some need less sleep than others. There is no norm for sleeping patterns in adults or children. If we expect a little less from our children in the way of set routines and long periods of sleep we would find it much easier to cope with.'

The association originally acted as a postnatal support group, issuing newsletters and giving members a chance to swop experiences and tips, but now limit themselves to providing leaflets. Some of the groups that were started to offer more immediate advice can be contacted through Cry-sis, who offer support for sleep problems as well as crying (see later).

Practical solutions offered by professionals and parents are varied, but close physical contact does seem to reduce wakefulness and limit the disruption. Taking the baby into a family bed and suckling it on demand has been the answer for many parents. However, it is realistic to expect infants to wake during the night – 40% still do so at one year. Babies' sleep patterns are different from adults and contain more rapid eye movement sleep from which they are easily woken. Accepting disturbed nights while they last can be much less physically and emotionally draining than fighting them and make it easier to settle the baby again quickly. It is very important for mothers to avoid building up a fury of resentment. It may not be possible to cure wakefulness or avoid being tired, but a change of attitude can reduce the tension and prevent despair and depression setting in.

Crying

'A baby crying – one who goes on and on whatever you do – is about the most shattering sound anybody can hear. You cannot ignore it. It is like a screwdriver in your gut and a sledgehammer pounding your brain. A child who cries like this makes many mothers have dreadful thoughts of baby battering,' says Sheila Kitzinger. She was involved in a *Parents* survey into crying babies and their effects on parents. Of 705 mothers who replied, 'a staggering 92% said that they spent up to 12 hours of every day on their own – often with a crying baby. It's not surprising that over half described feelings of desperation and over a third feelings of anger and depression.' The survey also found that 72% of babies started crying a lot during their first six weeks, while the Thomas Coram Research Unit found that daytime behaviour problems, especially crying ascribed to colic or feeding difficulties, was the most commonly mentioned problem up to seven weeks, reported by two-thirds of mothers. And the self-help group Cry-sis point out that approximately 10% of babies cry excessively.

Pat Gray, whose two babies both cried constantly, helped to set up Cry-sis in North London. Now they are a national network of local contact groups who aim to support emotionally the parents of babies who cry excessively and cause a great deal of disruption and concern to their parents. 'All members of Cry-sis have been through this experience and fully understand how frustrating and depressing a constantly crying baby can be. Often there is nothing physically wrong with the baby. We have found through our own experiences that parents feel alone with their problem, exhausted by the continual demands of the baby and worried by this apparently abnormal behaviour. The effects on the family, marriage and home, not to mention the relationship between mother and baby, can be catastrophic. Although there is provision in the health service for advising mothers with problems, we feel that in-depth support is generally lacking, due to the pressures of work on the health care professionals. We feel that we can share our experience and practical tips and we hope to be able to add constructively to the information available on the reasons for some babies being unsettled.'

Cry-sis receive referrals from health visitors, midwives and GPs, or are contacted directly by parents. The groups provide telephone and personal contact, trying to introduce women to each other, and emphasise the benefits of joining any mother and baby group. Cry-sis do not offer medical advice but can make available practical information on possible causes, which include breastfeeding problems, allergies and colic, and check that parents have consulted their doctor about the baby's constant crying.

Cry-sis and other groups advise a flexible approach, especially to sleeping arrangements. The La Leche League say, 'It is only when you have a baby of your own that you realise what a disturbing thing it is to hear a baby cry – not just any baby, but your baby. It makes mothers feel quite desperate.' They start a list of possible reasons for crying with 'Most of all your baby wants *you*. She wants your milk, your arms, your heartbeat, the sound and smell of you. You are her only source of nourishment, warmth, comfort, a reassuring sameness,' and suggest baby carriers as a way of comforting babies while getting other things done.

Often, because a mother is so desperate, tired and depressed, a doctor will prescribe drugs for her baby. Sheila Kitzinger says in *The Sunday Times*, 'By the time they are 18 months old, 25% of babies have already had sedatives, some for four months or more.' Most colic medicines are also central nervous system depressants, sedating the baby. Apart from the dangers of these drugs (some have been withdrawn from use for younger babies), side-effects often include making the baby miserable and irritable the next day. Sheila

Kitzinger is concerned about a further side-effect. 'Some babies are so heavily drugged that they no longer make eye contact with their mothers, have to be roused for feeds and then suck feebly before falling asleep again. . . These drug-stupefied babies are often unrewarding for their mothers,' and this loss of contact 'has serious consequences for the mother-child relationship.'

Alternatively, the baby's crying may be a response to its mother's irritability and lack of interest. She may already be depressed or distressed, and the baby's crying drives her further down the slope. The only way to break the cycle is to discover the real cause of the depression – nutritional, hormonal, events from the past surfacing, an emotional reaction to the birth, or present circumstances. During this time support is vital and all groups emphasise how important it is for someone else to take the baby for short periods.

One destructive emotion it is essential to help mothers get rid of is guilt. Mothers feel guilty because they cannot stop the baby crying, and because they resent the endless demands. Blaming the baby is the next stage, easily followed by hitting the baby. Being supported can restore a sense of proportion. As with wakefulness, if no solution can be found, realising that at least the baby will eventually settle down and accepting what is happening may be better than resisting and resenting, and take a lot of tension and bitterness out of the situation. Other mothers can also increase understanding of the baby's point of view. 'Crying is their only language, though for adults it can be the most difficult to learn,' says Sheila Kitzinger.

Allergies

Sensitivities to foods and environmental substances can affect mood and behaviour as well as producing physical symptoms (see Chapter 4). A mother can become exhausted, baffled and depressed dealing with a child who is irritable, fidgety, wakeful and cries a lot. Babies can react adversely to infant formulas based on cow's milk or soya, and to goat's milk. They may react to substances their mothers have eaten which are passed to them in their milk.

Why babies get colic, which causes them to scream, cry and refuse to be comforted, often for hours on end and usually in the evenings, for weeks and even months, is not known for sure. Some studies have found that cutting out cow's milk from the baby's or breastfeeding mother's diet, both as a drink and in foods, does stop the symptoms. Another study found that the effect of parental smoking on colic was 'striking'. When only the mother smoked, their infants had almost twice the incidence of colic (57%) as children of non-smokers (32%). Where the mother was a non-smoker but the father smoked more than 20 cigarettes a day, 91% of the babies got colic.

Cry-sis estimate that 40% of babies who cry excessively suffer from allergies. Sally Bunday's discoveries with her own crying baby, later a seriously hyperactive child, started her campaigning for the spread of information. At the time Miles was born Sally knew nothing about the links between chemicals in food and the environment and a baby's behaviour. Miles never stopped screaming, day and night, feeding took forever as he thrashed about, he hardly ever slept, and had to be strapped into his pram to stop him throwing himself out. And, like many children with allergies, he was endlessly thirsty (this itself can cause crying and wakefulness). Through years of impossible behaviour that caused her to lose weight and be permanently exhausted and unable to cope, plus totally disrupting the family's life and seriously straining her marriage, she was told nothing could be done and felt she was somehow to blame. Then, after finding information on diet and mental states and eliminating various chemicals from Miles's diet, his behaviour changed completely.

She now runs the Hyperactive Children's Support Group. They offer support, sometimes being a mother's last hope, plus information and practical advice. The earlier parents are aware of the possible role of allergies, the less likely it is they will get desperate. Knowing what to do can even avoid any allergic reaction in a potentially sensitive child. Breastfeeding up to about nine months and delaying the introduction of solids for as long as is practicable reduces the incidence of allergic reactions, as does reducing exposure to animals and house dust, household chemicals and environmental pollutants. But action can be taken even earlier. The pre-conceptual care group Foresight point out that sensitivities can start while the baby is in the womb so that a balanced diet of whole fresh foods and the avoidance of harmful substances by pregnant women helps to prevent problems in their babies.

When pregnancy goes wrong

Instead of pregnancy proceeding smoothly and producing a strong healthy baby, things can go unexpectedly wrong. When they do, it is inevitable that the mother will be very sad. Sometimes, because of physical shock to her system, the disruption of the usual pattern of hormonal changes during pregnancy and birth, the reactivation of earlier painful events, or the fact that her partner cannot adjust to whatever has happened to the baby and the relationship gets into difficulties or fails, natural healthy sorrow becomes clinical depression or puerperal psychosis.

Death of a baby, however soon after conception, requires mourning. If this process is suppressed or incomplete after the loss, the wound will always fester and the need to mourn will reappear later at a time of crisis or emotional vulnerability, such as the birth of a subsequent baby. Because deaths of full-term babies are unusual nowadays, family, friends and professional staff as well as the mother are stunned. Perhaps because death in a medical wonderworld has overtones of failure it may be rushed out of the way by everyone. Efforts are being made to change this and in miscarriage, stillbirth and perinatal deaths it is recognised that it is easier for the loss to be accepted as true, then grieved for, if the parents have an opportunity to see or hold the foetus or baby if they wish. The baby may be named and photographs taken. Requests for some kind of funeral ceremony to acknowledge the baby's brief life and mark and dignify its death are starting to be treated sympathetically.

No one plans what to do if they lose their baby, and shocked parents will be in no state to make arrangements, so support is vital, and subsequent counselling may be advisable. Self-help groups can assist in two ways. Members of general groups to which a mother already belongs can be with her quickly, perhaps supporting her through the miscarriage or stillbirth or immediately after the death. They are well placed to make early contact with groups like the Stillbirth and Neonatal Death Society. These groups can offer detailed information and skilled support.

Chris Burrows of the NCT says, 'What can a postnatal supporter do to help? First of all, try to understand what the mother's feelings are. They include shock, isolation, frustration, guilt and anger as well as sorrow. Shock, because she expected birth and life, and got death. Isolation, because from her point of view at least, all her friends seem to have a baby or be pregnant except her, and very few people understand her situation. Frustration, because mothering starts at birth, even when the baby is dead, and cannot be turned off like a tap.

'The physical discomforts of birth are still there: stitches for example, and the milk which comes in although there is no baby. The "empty arms" syndrome is no myth, and may even be felt as a physical ache. Guilt, because she may feel that something she did, or did not, do during pregnancy caused the baby's death . . . Anger, against her GP, the hospital staff, her husband or, most of all, herself for "letting it happen".'

She points out that recovery from the death of a baby takes many months, often years, and that mothers should not be expected to 'get over it' in a few weeks. All supporters emphasise that both parents need a chance to talk. NCT mother Sarah Playforth's son died when he was eight days old, but she has been able to come to terms with the loss. 'Had I not seen, held and known Benjamin, had I not grieved wholeheartedly, with the support of others, I would be bitter and unreconciled instead of occasionally very sorrowful, yet philosophical.'

Women who have had their pregnancies terminated, for whatever reason, may feel only enormous relief, or they may feel guilty and angry that this seemed the only decision they could make. If the termination is early in the pregnancy, unpleasant feelings may appear to go away quite quickly. Women who have later terminations, however, perhaps at five months after discovering through amniocentesis tests that their baby is handicapped, have to endure a traumatic physical process and their dead baby is much more real, so their disturbance is likely to be much greater. Whatever the stage that the pregnancy was terminated, and however well the mother adjusts at the time, feelings of guilt and grief can easily be awakened by a subsequent pregnancy. As with other forms of loss of a child, the mother may also confuse the identities of the two babies. Being able to talk about their feelings with other mothers is very important to women who have been through abortions.

Mothers have to cope with a mass of confused feelings, including grief and self-blame, when they discover their child is physically or mentally handicapped or ill in some way. Fortunately, there are now self-help groups to assist with almost all types of problem after birth. As well as campaigning for research, better information and more government aid, these groups supply a lot of practical help and advice, gathered firsthand, and help whole families adjust to what has happened. But, perhaps the most important way in which they sustain mothers and prevent them from becoming overwhelmed and depressed, is by banishing the sense of isolation that mothers of handicapped children suffer.

Now both premature and small-for-dates babies stand a greater chance of survival because of improved techniques of neonatal intensive care, although facilities vary from area to area and the Baby Life Support Systems group say organisation of care for very small or ill babies is 'inadequate, haphazard and unstructured'. Nearly one-fifth of all newborns will spend some of their first hours or days in a neonatal unit. For a woman to have her baby taken into special care is very distressing for a variety of reasons. She is worried about the baby's chances of survival or of becoming healthy or normal, she usually cannot breastfeed her baby and is deprived of holding, cuddling and caring for it and, if she goes home before the baby can, visiting may be a great strain on the whole family.

Some evaluation is being done into whether all babies that go into special care should be there, into less technological ways of getting fragile babies to thrive, such as carrying the baby next to the mother's breasts all the time, and routines within special care baby units are being questioned to see if closer contact between mother and baby is possible. It is now recognised that separation is harmful to mother and baby and to the bond between them. However, even if conditions change, some mothers will still have to cope with worries about their babies' welfare and the pain of being away from them. Again, the support of mothers who have been through the experience and have formed self-help groups is invaluable in stopping mothers with babies in special care becoming hopelessly depressed.

Caesarean section is on the increase (see Chapter 2). Whether babies born in this way need to go into special care or whether they are perfectly fit, mothers who have had caesarean sections are more likely to get PND than those who have not. The reasons for this may be partly physical – the trauma of surgery, the use of anaesthetics and disruption of the hormonal pattern during birth, plus pain, discomfort and restricted mobility. But it is clear that caesarean mothers have feelings of disappointment, failure, dissatisfaction, misunderstanding and worry that need to be voiced, sympathised with and worked through. The caesarean support groups that are being set up provide practical information and help, but they also help mothers to analyse unresolved issues that can cause depression sooner or later after the birth, and they can support or refer women who they realise are suffering from PND.

Stress and violence

A mother who is suffering from PND or who is exhausted or unhappy, has a low threshold of patience. Difficulties with her baby – feeding problems, wakefulness, crying, unsettled behaviour – can both worsen physical exhaustion and compound any emotional or psychological problems by causing guilt and resentment, and by making establishing a bond with the baby hard.

In this situation many mothers fear harming their babies, and some actually do lose control. In a *Parents* survey on crying babies nearly a quarter of mothers felt like smacking the baby and one in ten did so. Ill-treatment can vary from isolated incidents of rough handling, smacking or throwing the baby into its cot through spanking to, occasionally, severe beatings and downright torture. Most mothers feel deep self-loathing when they ill-treat their baby, even once in a very minor way, and lock the incident away, vowing never to repeat it. Fear of hurting the baby may be greater than the chances of anything actually happening again. But it is all too easy for loss of control to become an escalating pattern, especially if the baby becomes disturbed and manifests this through more crying, feeding difficulties or wakefulness.

The Pacific Post Partum Support Society found that when they examined the problems of women who came to them with PND, about 70% of the parents had problems related to their children, ranging from actual physical abuse to over-concern – often a manifestation of resentment and lack of feeling for a child. Joann Robertson, who helped set up the society and works for the prevention and treatment of child abuse and says, 'Child abuse, potential or active, is one manifestation of depression.' Mothers who seek professional help often run into a barrier. When they express their fears of killing or hurting their babies, or confess to actual violence, they are met with reassurances that these are symptoms of PND and that, of course, they will not really hurt their babies. If they confess to actual violence treatment is directed to curing the depression alone.

In talking of ways of helping these parents Joann Robertson says that parents fall into separate groups with different needs that can be responded to in different ways. The smallest, most clear-cut group have children who are so clearly at high risk they are likely to be taken into care. The second group may be resistant to help because of their fear and lack of trust. They are likely to have been emotionally or physically abused as children themselves. Family counselling is often needed here.

Self-motivated mothers who actively seek help are the most likely to have their needs brushed aside because they do not conform to stereotypes of abusive parents. It may be thought that they merely have unrealistic ideas about parenthood and require more information. But, 'Since many of these parents already know how to parent or know what kind of parent they want to be, the books and classes recommended simply increase their feelings of inadequacy, guilt and helplessness; it is their emotional response to the child which is the problem.'

Voluntary and self-help organisations play a vital role in averting or stopping child cruelty and assisting parents to deal with situations that could lead to violence. One mother who was very disturbed postnatally and whose baby was ill writes in the NCT magazine *New Generation* about ringing the National Society for the Prevention of Cruelty to Children, 'I was sure that soon I would hurt the child badly. I had already thrown him on the bed and was throwing other things about like a wild thing when he screamed . . . The treatment I received was quite literally life-saving. The local NSPCC inspector came *immediately*, telling me to put the baby in his cot and wait by the door for him to arrive. He stayed with me almost the whole day. He heard my distress. He sympathised with the problems of the baby's illness. He reassured me that I was going through a very harrowing time, that I was under an enormous strain, that I was not insane. He treated me as an intelligent equal. He visited me every week for about two months.'

A mother's total indifference to her baby that is one symptom or effect of PND can, as much as impatience, lead on to abuse. The NSPCC say they are 'very conscious of the effects of postnatal depression, not only in provoking abuse but in preventing the formation of those bonds between mother and child so essential for the child's future protection. We try to work closely with midwives, health visitors and other medical staff in alleviating it in the families we are helping.'

Many parents want to stay anonymous until they are confident enough to ask for professional advice, or find speaking with others who have fought their own ambivalent and aggressive feelings more helpful. Various groups reach parents under stress. Home-Start schemes around the country offer support, friendship and practical help to such parents and may be alerted by health visitors and social workers or PND support groups when mothers have PND. They work through individual volunteers and management teams who liaise with relevant voluntary groups and professionals. Organisations for Parents Under Stress is an umbrella name for a network of groups who give support and advice to parents under stress who may feel themselves and their children to be at risk. They usually work through a confidential telephone service. Stella Sherrat of OPUS says, 'The aim of the volunteer is to help the parent see things clearly. Our emotions are so closely linked with those of our children that the way through the entanglement of guilt and love, hate and worry is impossible without some outside non-directive counselling.' OPUS believe that isolation is one of the main stresses leading to child abuse and that this can be alleviated by encouraging parents to come together, to help each other grow and develop.

Stress and addiction

No one knows how many women seek escape from marital and postnatal problems through alcohol and drugs. Those who are already users may find the emotional stress of motherhood turns them into alcoholics or drug addicts, then that the practical demands of motherhood make kicking the habits nearly impossible.

One mother who started taking heroin after her son was born soon became addicted. 'Slowly everything turns around; you're not using heroin to get stoned, suddenly you need it to get up and cope with the baby. With kids it is hard to come off heroin – you don't have time to withdraw.' Her baby was taken into care for short periods. Scared she would lose him she tried detoxification twice but it was not until she got into Meta House, the only long-term residential house in the country that caters solely for women drug addicts, that she began to get the problem under control.

The staff at Meta House believe women use drugs to blot out feelings of worthlessness. Justine Picardie and Dorothy Wade, who wrote *Heroin: Chasing the Dragon*, say in *The Sunday Times* that women take drugs for different reasons from men. 'Women are far more likely to use drugs as a means of escape: from bad marriages, from problems of parenthood, from depression (the incidence of those who have become addicted to prescribed tranquillisers and then progress to illegal drugs is very high among women).'

Mothers face other problems in trying to give up drugs. 'Ironically, sometimes the reason for their addiction can also be the reason for their reluctance to come forward. For a mother, the greatest fear is that if she tells her doctor or a social worker of her addiction, her child will immediately be taken away and put into care. This fear is quite justified: the children of drug users are automatically put on the "At Risk" register.' When mothers do come forward, official resources for treating them without separating them from their children are almost non-existent, as is so with women alcoholics. Because of this, and because of the fear of losing their children, 'Instead women use covert means. According to a London survey, telephone helplines, self-help groups, advice agencies, particularly those staffed by women, are all popular means of support.'

Chapter 7

Helping yourself

In the end, no matter how much support you receive from other people, the only person who can decide how kindly you will be treated is yourself. You are the only person who can define your feelings, choose your attitudes, what compromises you will or will not make, and what risks you will take. It is up to you to determine what you are prepared to put up with as an individual woman and as a representative of one half of the population.

Emotional and physical disturbances in the postnatal period originate in stress and exhaustion. If you decide that your own well-being in this period is essential, not only to your future mental and physical health but for the best interests of your baby, any older children and your partner, it is possible to reduce much stress and put yourself in good shape to cope with what is unavoidable. There are many ways of taking care of yourself, both in the senses of nurturance and of protection. Attitudes as well as action are important. You need to be positive in not just letting things happen to you, and in being sure that you do not view birth, motherhood, unpredictable emotions and even depression in a negative light.

Finally, if you want children you must accept that it is time to grow up. Maturation is not finite but continuous, if uneven. Whether you manage to take major steps to maturity before you become pregnant, during the birth or soon afterwards, gradually over the following months, or not until well into your baby's childhood, could be critical in determining how likely or not you are to succumb to PND.

TAKE CARE OF YOURSELF

However many demands seem to be placed on a new mother, and however little time and energy she feels she has for herself, the situation can usually be made more favourable by a careful choice of priorities. Assuming that partners give as much as they take (an ideal form of relationship but one that can and does exist), and that a return to paid work is not immediate, the following would be a sensible order for dealing with responsiblities.

THE RIGHT PRIORITIES

- *welfare of the baby and other children* – basic needs do not include spotless clothes and mothers are not the only people who can supply children's needs
- *welfare of the mother* – it is not going to help anyone if mothers make no provision for their physical, mental, emotional and spiritual needs and so become ill
- *domestic tasks* – regular good food is vital for all the family; everything else can be put in a descending order of importance (it is amazing how many household jobs can wait one to five years to be done)

Looking after children

Children are dependent and their needs have to come first, however drained a mother feels, but there is no merit in turning yourself into a martyr, let alone reaching the stage where you cannot function. Partners and anyone who exhibits or can be persuaded to take an interest in the baby should be enrolled to lighten the load. Many mothers have a total block about sharing or delegating any tasks or care. It is probably true that it is simpler for others to help with domestic tasks, freeing mothers to care for their infants, especially if they are breastfed, but it is worth looking carefully at every offer of assistance. One way of getting time to catch up or, better, time to rest is to share childcare with other mothers, one mother taking two babies while one mother has a break.

Attitudes to children are examined in the second half of this chapter while special needs – coping with breastfeeding, wakefulness, crying, allergies, handicap and illhealth – are dealt with in Chapter 6 and Getting Help. Whatever the problem, major or minor, an open mind and flexible approach defuses the tension, resentment and anger that can lead on to depression. The Association of Breast-feeding Mothers offer this advice, to be applied to all manner of problems. 'Don't reject any suggestion once and for all; as your baby grows you may find a different approach to the problem offers a more satisfactory solution.'

Being kind to yourself

Women find it hard to take care of themselves – because of real pressures on their time and energy, but also because they often feel they do not have a right to much consideration, from themselves or others, and they believe that being womanly means putting others first all the time. The roots of these attitudes and alternative ways of looking at ourselves are considered in Chapter 3 and later in this chapter.

Once a woman has sunk into PND she will find it very hard to muster the enthusiasm and self-esteem to help herself in any way, which is why support from her partner and other women is so vital (see Chapter 6). But after she has been persuaded that she is of value and entitled to consideration, she has to start the job of learning to be kind to herself in every way. This, and the whole process of arresting depression or recovering from it, is best done by taking one day at a time, setting extremely modest goals and doing things little by little.

YOUR PHYSICAL HEALTH

This is a prime consideration in avoiding or limiting PND. The following will all reduce stress and increase resistance to it, so lessening the chances of deep fatigue and depression.

- getting adequate rest
- regularly eating sufficient nutritious food
- going outdoors every day
- taking exercise
- following relaxation techniques
- going to singing or dancing classes
- taking short breaks away from the home (and, perhaps, the family)

It is true that many mothers, even when they simplify their lives and responsibilities as far as they can, have little time left for their physical health. The above list is, therefore, impossible for most mothers to follow in every point, but it has a value as a state of affairs to aim for, and as a checklist to see if you are doing *any one* of these things to care for your health.

BREATHE

b reathe deeply to relieve tension, frustration and anger.

r elax for 15 minutes each day. Seek out a quiet place to relieve stress.

e xercise regularly each day. Very important for reducing toxins in the blood, when we get upset. Walking has been found invaluable in coping with depression. Gentle exercise for a few minutes every day.

a ccept your depression. Seeking instant recovery, will lead to more anxiety and depression. Your depression is telling you that there is something wrong with the way you are living.

t herapy. Share your problems with someone, talk about them.

h ealthy diet. Avoid junk foods, reduce tea, coffee and alcohol which are all depressants. Avoid white sugar, white bread, white flour. Increase intake of fresh vegetables and fruit.

e nterprise. Set yourself a challenge. To overcome your depression take up some creative activity: drawing, painting, etc.

Suggestions for taking care of yourself and dealing with depression by Shirley Toms

---

Running the home

Surrounded by advertising telling them how easy it is to have a beautiful well-kept home, many women attempt to keep up domestic standards that are quite unrealistic for one person to achieve, especially if she has a paid job as well as being a mother. In the bad old days women who prized their image as a good housewife were frequently managers of servants. Poorer women had less of everything so stuck to basic tasks. Either way, no one had any illusions about housework being time-consuming. Nowadays, women have to learn to resist pressures to be superwoman (see Chapter 3). This is not too difficult a task if you decide firmly that you value your health, happiness and sanity more than other people's opinions, and that you will play your part in putting paid to this silly circle of housewifely oneupmanship. If you feel your family must come first, ask yourself what really contributes to their welfare – an orderly dust-free house or shared time and laughter?

The Association of Breastfeeding Mothers have crammed more sensible advice into one Handy Hints leaflet than most officially funded or commercial bodies manage in their larger, glossier publications. The leaflet places people firmly before things but recognises that the home still has to function and offers some helpful pointers.

Taking care

Pregnancy is not a time to be heroic, nor are the first few months after baby's arrival. Avoid altogether heavy work. This may seem obvious, but we can sometimes feel very awkward about refusing to assist. A lot of babies have been weaned because people try to move house, take foreign holidays and carry out other strenuous projects in the first six months. After a difficult birth, like a caesarean section, it would be sensible to avoid all that for a year if at all possible.

Planning ahead

Pregnancy is a good time for thinking about values and deciding what's really important. Be selective about getting unfinished projects done before the baby comes. Organise any repairs and maintenance work on your house/car/washing machine or whatever you consider essential. Think in terms of minimising the work you will be doing later. For example, a washing machine and a secondhand pram would make more sense than endless trips to the launderette with an expensive new pram.

Clear the decks

Pregnancy is also a time to simplify – go through the house and give as much to the jumble sale as you can. Fiddly things that need to be ironed/dusted/polished can be put away in boxes and stored. Once you start thinking in terms of 'Do I really need to do this?' it is surprising how much turns out to be non-essential.

Shopping

Stock up while you are pregnant – a freezer is a great help. In the early weeks order by phone whenever you can. When you go out be prepared for disasters you could ordinarily handle, but which under the circumstances would be too much. If anyone will help with shopping and general chores, let them.

Housework

Take pride in your family and not in your house. Look at nursing your baby as a time to rest. If you have other children this is a golden opportunity to spend time with them as well. If you cannot stand the mess, try concentrating on one room at a time. The kitchen and bathroom are the only rooms that really need to be clean. Delegate chores to other members of the family. The chaos is only temporary.

Feeding yourself

Make sure you get three to four meals a day. These do not all have to be cooked but can be simple foods with high nutritional value. Preparing the evening meal partly in the morning when you have more energy and time could make all the difference. Casseroles are a lifesaver and you may find a slow cooker would be a good investment.

Taking steps to make life easier, and enrol help from partners and others, would seem a straightforward thing to do, but a lot of mothers have blocks about sharing their domestic role, even when they are doing fulltime paid work. Terri Apter, author of *Why Women Don't Have Wives: Professional Success and Motherhood*, writing in *Cosmopolitan* says, 'Women think if they are to have everything – husband, children and work – just as a man, then they must do everything, *unlike* a man.' Women may, through aptitude or social influence, be better at nurturing, but that is no reason why all domestic jobs should be left to women. It does mean that 'women will have to work a little harder to get the help they need from husbands and fathers. They will have to develop another skill – that of learning how to teach their men about wifely roles. This means, too, that women will have to relinquish some of that special pride and pleasure in always being the best when it comes to domesticity. They will have to *accept* help in the home, as well as *giving* it.' But if women are to become good at teaching partners and fathers how to share the job of wife they need to become mature enough to see 'the illogic of thinking only of helping others, and the inequality of always making sacrifices for or protecting someone else.'

Ways of altering mood

Paying attention to health factors has an additional and specific value in relation to PND because there are ways of directly or indirectly altering metabolism and brain chemistry and so mood – in the short or longer term. (For fatigue see Chapter 3; nutrition Chapter 4.)

Exercise

This speeds up metabolism and improves mood. Walking, running, dancing and swimming can actually lift feelings of depression. In a recent Norwegian study on the value of aerobic exercise in alleviating depression, it was shown that even a moderate increase in maximum oxygen intake (15–30%) had an antidepressive effect, and this occurred regardless of the severity of the depression.

Going out for regular exercise when you are looking after a new baby is often impossible, and many mothers who have worked-out religiously through their pregnancy stop completely after the baby is born. The only short-term answer may be to force yourself to do 10-minute stints of exercises when you can, throughout the day, dance to the radio when you can, plus take the baby out for a walk once a day, regardless of weather.

Music

We experience music through vibrations and vibrations affect mood and behaviour. It is possible to use music therapeutically in two ways. By listening to lively, cheerful, escapist music to cheer yourself up and, if possible, to encourage you into dancing or singing. Or by choosing profound and maybe very sad music to trigger you into a release of emotion and tears when you feel quite numb and cannot respond to anything, even your baby.

Dealing with tension

Mental and physical tension are a vital response to a stressful emergency, but when they persist they stop the body normalising all its functions again. The mood goes from a healthy alertness to chronic anxiety and, eventually, to clinical depression. 'Learning to relax' sounds a contradiction in terms, but certain techniques cut through the destructive circle of messages the body is sending itself. These techniques are best used as a preventative measure, to stop tension ever getting a hold, or to release it in the early stages before major mood changes become established. It is harder for someone who is depressed to use these techniques, but they can work.

Physical relaxation

All the methods affect mind and body, but some emphasise one over the other. Some of the simplest modern physical routines are based on the premise that, because of the way our reflexes are conditioned and the importance we place on language, you can take a short cut to relaxation by simply talking to your body. Say to your arms, 'Let go, let go, let go,' and they go limp. There are innumerable variations on this system, and one seems as effective as another.

The great art of hatha yoga (union by bodily control) aims to completely harmonise body, mind and soul. It is a path whose ultimate aim is bliss and ecstasy and its correct practice unquestionably restores and develops mental tranquillity and strength. It can easily be followed in the simplest form by a beginner who is not looking for spiritual insights, when its brilliantly devised exercises will still aid the body to achieve biochemical balance.

Breathing

Breathing deeply relieves frustration, anger and physical tension by causing biochemical alterations. An awareness of the key role of breathing to all forms of relaxation, and of gaining control by the mind over bodily functioning, is one immense gift of yoga. Most breathing exercises, including those used in childbirth, are derived from yoga breathing. Unfortunately, they have often become harmfully debased. Breathing awareness, not rigid control, is the true aim, and anything forced is counterproductive. Strained holding of the breath during birth is dangerous as the body is deprived of oxygen. One simple way of cutting short the panic or blind, hair-trigger anger that can be experienced postnatally is to breathe in slowly, counting to five, and out again, counting to 10, until you feel calm again.

Mental relaxation

Awareness of breathing is an important part of the ancient practice of meditation. The aim is to allow the mind to become completely still and its original purpose was spiritual enlightenment. Once this level of 'non-thinking' happens, it brings feelings of relaxation, detachment, calm and happiness. Energy, creativity and bliss well up and, afterwards, meditators feel refreshed and renewed. All these mental changes are accompanied by beneficial biochemical changes. There are many simple, non-religious forms of this practice which some people find more to their taste and easier to follow.

Complementary medicine

Most forms of complementary or alternative medicine approach mind and body holistically and are of value in preventing mild symptoms deteriorating into serious ill-health – physical or mental. The aim is to assist the body in helping itself, to stimulate or strengthen its own mechanisms for re-establishing equilibrium. Many of the therapies can be used to treat a woman who has PND, either by dealing with a particular physical problem so that her energies can be given wholly to recovery from depression, or by improving her general health. But some have a good reputation for dealing with anxiety and depression more directly.

The Alexander technique

'A way of becoming more aware of balance, posture and movement in everyday activities, this can bring into consciousness tensions previously unnoticed, and helps us differentiate between necessary and unnecessary (appropriate and inappropriate) tensions and effort.' The links between tension and depression have already been discussed. As this technique requires personal tuition over three to five months, it is most valuable taken up in early pregnancy. It is of great assistance in knowing how to make active uses of the body during labour and birth, so lessening the chances of distressing interventions (see Chapter 2).

Cranial osteopathy

Through touching and gentle manipulation of the bones of the head and upper spine, cranial osteopaths can assess the state of connective tissue throughout the body and restore its proper functioning where necessary. They can prepare pregnant women for an easier birth by making the pelvis more mobile and tissue more elastic. They believe PND is caused by downward displacement of the womb during birth, and a resultant tug on the pituitary gland via the covering of the spinal cord and brain. They expect treatment for PND to work within two weeks.

Herbal medicine

The orthodox medical view has been that this is unscientific and ineffectual, but clients have been satisfied with the help herbalists have given them. Now these traditional remedies are being attacked as dangerous and there is pressure for them to be subject to analysis and rigorous tests. Tony Hampson, joint chairman of the Natural Medicines Group, says, 'Practitioners of natural medicine accept that it is the whole plant in harmony which provides the remedy not just the active principle. This element of harmony is part of the philosophy of holistic medicine.' Meanwhile, it is still possible to obtain a wide variety of plant substances with a proven history of relieving tension, of stimulating mood, or lifting depression.

Homoeopathy

The philosophy of this therapy is to provide a natural healing process, 'using remedies that assist the patient to regain health by stimulating the body's own powers of recovery.' It treats the whole person, not symptoms in isolation, and treats the patient rather than the disease. Because the remedies are prescribed on an individual basis, no single one is used for PND. Instead, a choice is made from a wide range of substances derived from vegetable, animal and mineral sources, according to personality type and what is thought to have caused the depression. Homoeopaths also believe that when parents or more remote forbearers have been victims of major infectious diseases, such as tuberculosis, a resulting biochemical imbalance can be inherited, including an endocrine imbalance. These individuals would then be especially susceptible to PND.

Lists of practitioners, reading lists and general information on complementary therapies are available from the relevant professional bodies.

Learning what you can

Professional opinion is divided as to whether it is possible or desirable to teach people how to prepare themselves for marriage or parenthood, because the experiences and ways of dealing with them that are presented may bear little relation to what happens to a particular couple in partnership or parenthood and, if they run into problems, this disparity could be an added source of stress. It is also possible that the teachers could be offering notions that are, in their own way, as unrealistic as any held by those being instructed.

Part of the motivation to prepare parents, especially mothers, for parenthood comes from ideas that the arrival of a first child creates a crisis for the couple, and that motherhood is a maturational crisis (see chapter 3). This has led to attempts to prepare the parents psychologically and emotionally as well as at a practical level for the arrival of their baby. Some studies have moderated this perception, for example 'it is more accurate to think of beginning parenthood as a transition accompanied by some difficulty, than a crisis of severe proportions' (Hobbs and Cole 1976). Other authorities have argued against any blanket approach on the basis that pregnant women and new mothers vary in their psychological state as much as any other women. In a chapter on pregnancy and after in *Contributions to Medical Psychology* Dr Sandra Elliott says '. . . there is no evidence that all pregnant women, or expectant couples, require psychotherapy. Rather they would benefit from practical advice on preparing their physical and social environment for their new life style with a (another) child . . .'

When information about what can happen between two partners and their children is put forward in a non-directive way as possibilities and options it does seem to help parents to have more realistic expectations about each other, the birth, and the baby. Christopher Clulow of the Institute of Marital Studies in one project found that couples resisted knowledge that would 'upset' their ideas. This finding could provide an argument against parents' attending classes. Reading books on marital relationships, birth, parenting and child development would be less threatening ways of meeting new knowledge and ideas than coming face to face with some authoritative figure. Readers can take everything at their own pace, put books down when they become boring or disturbing, go back again later. No loss of face is involved in changing ideas as a result of what has been read.

Talking with trusted friends who have gone through similiar experiences or difficulties (and possibly changed their views as a result), plus handling their children, are good ways of learning more. The Thomas Coram Research Unit found that women who had had most to do with babies before their pregnancy were less likely to say

245

they were coping with difficulty and drew the conclusion that 'such prior dealings may give some parents more confidence and skill in early dealings with their new child.'

Learning about PND from any sources – what can cause it, its symptoms and various forms – may not prevent it starting but can enable a mother and her partner to recognise quickly what is going wrong and act to contain it. If it runs its course (see later), at least they know what is happening and that it will end, which takes the panic, fear and hopelessness out of the situation.

TAKING STEPS TO REDUCE STRESSES

The more you learn about what can contribute to PND, the more steps you can take to eliminate or reduce stressful factors.

- *get informed*: the greater your knowledge about dealing with small babies, the simpler it will be
- *accept help* from your partner, relatives, neighbours, friends
- *establish links* with other couples who have small children
- *do not move* home while the baby is tiny; try to stay put during pregnancy and the first year
- *choose priority tasks* and let everything else slide
- *rest* as much as you can; learn to catnap
- *shed responsibilities* for others wherever you can
- *cut down* on demanding outside activities, but do not become a hermit
- *communicate* your fears, worries and plans to your partner and those who are close to you
- *arrange babysitting* care; make it reciprocal if you cannot afford to pay
- *get to know* your GP, health visitor and clinic, if possible

---

Working for change

A contribution to reducing depression after birth can be made by working to reduce the sources of stress on mothers. Each woman could, from the time she plans to have children, concentrate on considering carefully what causes stress in her own life. But, once aware that most aspects of childbearing could be different, and better, most women find themselves involved in making efforts to change things for other mothers, too, and, in the long term, for their own children.

The areas in which change is desirable or possible are listed below, grouped under the headings of the chapters of this book in which they have been considered.

1 *Professional awareness of PND*
   recognition of the scale of PND
   accurate definitions
   increased understanding of origins
   improved ways of treating
2 *Birth*
   changes in organisation of NHS care antenatally, during birth and postnatally
   respect accorded to women's wishes by the medical profession
3 *Relationships and social conditions*
   equality of social and economic conditions for women
   improved status of motherhood
   availability of realistic information on partnership and parenthood
   more and better services/facilities for mothers/young children
   increased child benefit
   improved parental leave
   better childcare arrangements for working parents
   flexible working arrangements for women and men
4 *Biochemical factors*
   recognition of the role of hormones and nutrition
   availability of better information on diet
   prevention of adulteration of food and pollution of the environment
   subsidies, where necessary, to provide high-quality food for mothers
5 *Mental health care*
   woman-orientated perspectives in psychotherapy
   decreased dependence on drugs and ECT
   respect accorded to women by mental health care professionals

6 *Community awareness of PND*
greater communication between partners and with other individuals
improved status for self-help groups
7 *Mothers' attitudes*
increased self-respect and self-awareness in mothers
acceptance of positive value of children and their place in the community
acceptance of depression as something to be lived through and learned from

It is in the interests of women to work for improvements – not just from an altruistic point of view, but because they could be improving the situation for the time when they become mothers, or at least be better informed how to get the help or treatment they want during birth, soon afterwards, and as their children grow, or to protect themselves and their babies if necessary.

It is important that each and every mother recognises and accepts for herself how stressful motherhood can be, and that she makes it known to society in general so that there comes to be a better public recognition and acceptance of what motherhood involves, and mothers and small children are re-integrated back into the centre of society instead of being surrounded by a *cordon sanitaire* of attitudes and practical barriers as is often presently the case. If mothers do not consciously acknowledge that motherhood is hard, if rewarding, work, and blame themselves for finding it difficult to cope, the always destructive emotion of guilt will take hold. And by keeping their problems to themselves mothers fail to attract the support – from individuals or systems – to which they are entitled if society is sincere about regarding caring for children as an investment in everyone's future.

Some stresses are an inherent part of rearing children; others could and should be reduced or eliminated. Unavoidable stresses are a degree of physical tiredness, coping with the baby's ever-present total dependency, and working through the maturational process of becoming a mother. Stresses that society should strive to deal with are those resulting from conditions open to improvement which are listed earlier.

The list of established interests that mothers need to influence, educate or confront is formidable and few women, even if they have an overview and see links between them, will have the strength or time to work on all fronts. But anyone who needs reassurance about their right to stand up to paternalism or authoritarianism in health care and connected areas – those who insist they know what is good for us – has some heavyweight support. The World Health Organisation Alma Ata Declaration states, 'the people have a right and duty to participate in the planning and implementation of their own health care.'

Changing attitudes is a massive and slow task, but health care and support services are paid for by us all through our taxes and run, at some point, by elected or accountable individuals. Deciding how these services and policies could change to better serve a community's needs is down to us all. After studying first-time parents the Thomas Coram Research Unit offered a specification for a set of needs that services and policies affecting those making the transition to parenthood should be designed to meet. The needs were:

- for choice
- for information
- to discuss anxieties and feelings
- for effective help with child health and child management problems
- for adequate material and environmental conditions

Services dealing with pregnant women and mothers of small children are fragmented and uneven, yet co-ordination could pay dividends in preventing or picking up problems in mothers and babies. Realistic preparation for parenthood plus social support for new mothers could well result in fewer mothers with PND. Co-ordination could lead to a better understanding of needs and resulting changes in social policy. None of these improvements will happen if mothers individualise their difficulties and keep them secret.

The need for changes, and the role women have in achieving them, has been considered by the Boston Women's Health Book Collective. Some of the changes they suggest are:

- adequate subsidies for the diet of pregnant and postpartum women
- timely help for women who are likely to be upset postpartum
- groups for expectant parents to explore feelings and to provide instruction

- prenatal and postnatal hotline telephone services set up and staffed by women
- more females in obstetrics and gynaecology
- safe home delivery for those who want it
- paid maternity and paternity leave
- good childcare facilities

Self-transformation

As well as trying to see that society and its organisations constantly adapt to serve our needs – achieving change without – women can alter their perspectives and become more integrated and effective individuals through raising their consciousness and learning new skills – achieving change within.

Recognition by women that their situation is quite different from that of men, and that they need space, time, privacy and a sympathetic atmosphere to explore and consider themselves, the way they relate to other human beings and the way society is structured, has led to a growth in groups, classes and publications exclusively for women. Initial consideration often leads to asking questions and the realisation that they are short of knowledge – about everyday practicalities such as computer technology, car mechanics and tax regulations, or about the history and psychology of women.

Exploration can be both educational and therapeutic. It can remove blocks, untangle knots, increase maturity and confidence. It is easier to cope with birth and with motherhood if you have gone some way down the road to feeling optimistic, self-assured, mentally and physically fit, plus knowing who you are, what you want out of life and what price you are prepared to pay for it. Any reading material, gatherings or courses that aim at self-actualisation, and help a woman to gain strength and insight, will make motherhood happier and more rewarding and decrease the chances of emotional and mental disturbance after birth. Because the process of promoting personal growth takes time and energy, and because changes may occur slowly, it obviously would be more advantageous to start way back before planning a family, perhaps before entering a committed relationship. But it is not possible to plan life so neatly and mostly we must grow how and when we can, snatching opportunities as they are presented to us.

Certain information and techniques can lead to women gaining a completely new perspective on themselves and their place in society and contribute a lot to their maturation. Because of the commitment involved a mother who was deeply disturbed or depressed would inevitably find most of these activities too demanding, but mothers with milder PND could benefit – sometimes quite quickly. Although it takes a long time for all the seeds planted by reading a book or going to classes to come to full fruition, changes may be noticeable weeks, days, sometimes only hours after a particular point has registered. The sort of areas that can lead to self-transformation, and help protect against or lift depression are:

- co-counselling
- self-help group therapy
- consciousness raising
- women's studies
- assertiveness training
- women's self-defence
- martial arts
- singing
- dancing
- sport
- painting
- writing
- reading
- acquisition of new skills

Self-defence and self-assertion are key trainings to undertake because both require a woman to first take the step of deciding she is of value, that her value is being ignored, and that she wishes to change this. She can then go on to acquire techniques for defending her body and her whole person, making her presence felt and her wishes known in low-key but effective ways. Both types of training are based on a belief that women have the mental and physical resources to take care of themselves and ask for what is due to them, and aim to put women back in touch with these resources and develop them further.

COPING WITH YOUR FEELINGS

The Pacific Post Partum Support Society in Vancouver (see Chapter 6) have produced the following suggestions for women who feel tense, angry, stressed, depressed or disturbed after having a baby. This material also appears in the NCT booklet on PND – further evidence that women who know about PND have found the ideas useful and helpful. Some of the suggestions are for practical things to do, but what is really being put forward is an approach to coping with your feelings.

Dealing with anger and stress
Feelings of anger generally play an active part in depression. It is essential to get bottled-up anger 'out'. Otherwise, tension and stress can build, adding to the depression, completing a vicious circle. It is common for angry feelings to be directed at those closest to you, ie your husband or children; or at yourself. The following suggestions can help you to 'get rid' of the stress and tension caused by the angry feelings.

Physical expressions of anger
You may have the desire to express your anger in a physical way. When this happens, be sure that your child/ren are in a safe place, then try one or some of the following ideas. (The important thing to remember about these suggestions is that they are just that – suggestions. Try them all until you find one that you feel comfortable with and use it. Don't try one and feel that it is not working and not try the rest; *or* invent your own method for dealing with anger. You will know best what works for you.)

Getting the anger out
- Pound the counter, floor, wall, table.
- Tear up magazines or newspapers or old clothing.
- Break something, glasses, jars, bottles, etc (preferably in a paper bag, box etc, so that broken pieces will not have to be cleaned up).
- Pound a pillow, (this is much quieter than the above, especially if you live in an apartment or basement suite).
- Scream (into a pillow or out loud in a car), or cry. (If in a car you may need to pull over to the side of the road, as it may be scary to keep driving.)

- Skip rope (very fast).
- Run up and down a flight of stairs.
- Stamp your feet.
- Run around the outside of the house.
- Slam a door repeatedly.
- Lock yourself in the bathroom and slap a towel against the counter, wring a towel or bite it. (The bathroom is often the only place to have some privacy with your anger!)
- Call your volunteer or any person or place you feel you can trust, eg, neighbour, doctor, crisis centre, etc. It is important to talk about how you are feeling.

Calming down
- Wash your face with cold water.
- Turn on the shower and get in.
- Make a cup of tea or coffee, anything you find calming.

Verbal expressions of anger
You may find your anger coming out in verbal ways: eg yelling at children; or you may find yourself unable to talk to your partner without screaming when angry. Try yelling the things you wanted to say into a pillow, or in a closed room or car where others are unable to hear you. (It is often inhibiting to yell around others, therefore, the car or closed room.) You may also find it helpful to try some of the alternatives listed as physical actions.

Obsessive thinking and fantasies
For example: you may be thinking obsessively about death or illness; or you may be 'haunted' by an unpleasant experience (eg difficult labour and/or delivery or some other past experience which was hurtful to you). You could possibly be thinking a great deal about harming your child (either accidentally or purposely). For any of the above: don't try to control these thoughts – this will only make you more anxious and this in turn will increase the amount of destructive thinking you are doing. Get involved in activities that use large muscles (such as your arms and legs). Walk, do deep breathing, or anything that will help you to relax. Talk it over with your volunteer. Thoughts or fantasies do not have to be followed by action, nor is a fantasy the same as action. We have noticed that fantasies tend to become worse when you are tired. It is essential that you try to get plenty of rest.

Physical or emotional exhaustion

You may find yourself unable to touch or handle your children. You may have no feeling for the people in your life who are close to you or may be afraid of close emotional involvement. Some degree of this is completely normal at this time as it is such a draining time for you. You are constantly having to 'give' and care for others and there comes a point when you have to emotionally 'turn off'.

In any of these situations try to use babysitters as much as possible. Give yourself some time away from your family. It is very hard and wearing to be a 24-hour mother. In the beginning, taking time off can be difficult as you will probably feel guilty. If the feeling of guilt is there, try leaving the child for half an hour or an hour until you feel comfortable with that length of time and then try increasing it gradually. Do only what feels comfortable for you. When you have this time, we recommend that you try to do something for yourself, something that you used to like doing, that you haven't done for a long time. Some of these things are: going to museums or the library, window shopping, having coffee or lunch alone with a friend, taking a course or class or getting a babysitter to take the child to her home so that you can take that time to relax at home or sleep. (Whatever feels good.)

General tips

- Try to get enough sleep and watch that you are eating properly and regularly.
- You could try asking yourself some questions like, who or what am I really angry or resentful at.
- It is often very helpful to write down your feelings and perhaps look at them again when you are feeling calmer. In all cases – trust your feelings. Do not try to tell yourself, 'I shouldn't be angry.'
- If your angry feelings are frightening you, please share your thoughts with a safe person who will not judge you. You are not alone in having these feelings, nor are you a bad person for having them. It is important to discover ways to express them in a way that won't have negative repercussions in your life, but will help you to regain control.

Pacific Post Partum Support Society

THINK POSITIVE

The first section of this chapter dealt with things mothers can do for themselves to help avoid PND or limit its severity. But the way you think about your partner and children and what happens to you is another area of choice. Negative views sap energy and increase stress. They turn every life event into a problem, whereas seeing meaning and the possibility of growth in difficulties and disturbances can favourably influence the outcome.

Perhaps the greatest barrier to mothers seeing the postnatal period in a positive light, as a time when insights and strength can be gained through experiencing powerful, sometimes confusing emotions, is society's general fear of getting back in touch with the elemental. In the modern world birth may be the only time any of us comes so close to the grandeur and glory of nature. Women who open themselves to the experience of birth and motherhood are struck by a vision. Perhaps they do not know what to make of it, or how to communicate it. But while they struggle to do this, instead of being helped, the vision is denied. In particular, those who are involved in health care urge mothers to return quickly to 'normal' and feel compelled to treat mothers who do not do so. A greater respect for the changes of the postnatal period would be a contribution to society's positive thinking, but in the meantime it is open to you to change your individual perceptions.

Dealing with PND

Once you realise you are suffering from postnatal depression, however dispirited and demoralised you are there are still things you can do to help yourself – mainly by altering your view of what is happening to you. First you have to accept that there is a lot of thinking and understanding to be done before a 'cure' will result. You may choose to take drugs and undergo a course of ECT in the belief that this will lessen your symptoms and help you to cope with life and your baby again. These treatments may alleviate your symptoms, but you will still have to think about how to prevent yourself relapsing, why you got PND, and the meaning of the experience.

The easiest way to overcome the sensation that doing anything is overwhelmingly impossible and absolutely pointless is to break everything down into manageable parts. 'The question is not how to get cured, the question is how to live,' said writer Joseph Conrad. Postponing the question of how to get better and concentrating on how to survive makes more economic use of the energy you do have left. Settling for improvements 'one day at a time' will be more productive than having longer term plans and hopes. And breaking down the confusion of feelings that is attacking you into component parts makes it clearer where the roots of the individual feelings lie.

In their booklet *You Are Not Alone: Post-Natal Depression* Depressives Associated deal with two key emotions – anger (often unrecognised or unacknowledged) and guilt. Their attribution of the source of anger bears out the idea that depression is really a cry for love. 'When we are depressed, we often feel very angry. Sometimes for no apparent reason. It is common to direct these feelings of anger at those closest to us, the child(ren), our husband or relatives, our friends (those trying to help) and even ourselves. Again, such anger leads to feelings of guilt, so it becomes all too easy to believe that "they would be better off without me". *This is not true.*

'The anger you feel is a direct result of the pain you feel inside: the feeling that no-one understands or cares; the pain of rejection. The belief that you cannot go on, or cope any longer, is also the result of the emptiness you feel, the feeling that "this is never going to end". In time, with support, company that you find reassuring and care, the pain and emptiness will become less intense and you will discover that you *can* manage, that your concentration is improving and you are actually beginning to enjoy some aspect of your life!

'It is so important to remember that the pain, the emptiness, the anger, will not *always* overwhelm you, even though, at times, this seems to be so. The unpleasant feelings *will* go. One day, you will look back to discover that you have been feeling a little better . . .' The booklet emphasises how important it is to vent that anger harmlessly.

One DA newsletter recommends living in the present, not the painful past or the fearful future. The mind calms down miraculously and a lot of tension is dissipated when you purposely limit your frontiers to one day – today. Simplifying life in this way is vital. 'Depression is telling us that we need to slow down: our minds and our bodies.' Speaking our thoughts to ourselves or putting them on paper forces the mind to slow down. 'Rest your body also. Do not feel guilty if you lack energy or motivation. Rest. That's what the depression is telling you to do . . . We cannot do the things we would normally. So what? They will just have to wait for a while! When you are ready, tackle the smaller and "less pleasant" tasks first. One at a time. If it's a large task, do some now. Do some later. One step at a time. And you *will* get better. Not overnight. In time. Be patient with yourself and others . . . Be gentle with yourself.'

Very small shifts in attitude can turn the impossible into the possible. We need to realise that we do have resources and choices. 'We really do have a choice. No matter how much our illness tries to convince us "it is hopeless" we can choose the positive and devise little ways to keep the destructive thoughts from coming in.' No matter how limited our resources appear to be there is a way to use them effectively if we stop going round in circles of negative thought.

Although you know you feel low, unhappy and disturbed you may decide you are not suffering from PND but going through a difficult stage in your life. You may then feel that you want to work things out for yourself and that the professionals you have seen are giving answers that are wrong for you – because you do not agree with what they are saying or the treatment they are suggesting or because they are hurrying you to get better.

Understanding necessitates making connections. To have a hypothesis to test about your emotional functioning involves making speculative connections. These may be wrong, but you will never find the right set of connections if you do not cast around, putting forward and examining apparently untenable, unrealistic, uncomfortable, even bizarre ideas. There is no reason why your speculations about the origins of your PND should be less fruitful than an outsider's, however expert. So, if you think you might be on the track of working out what is going wrong in your life – things dating from your past, your present circumstances, or even your biochemical functioning – try trusting yourself and putting your theories to the test. If they are wrong you will have to have the courage to go on seeking answers.

In childbearing and in mental distress there is a failure on the part of individuals to take charge of their lives and a failure on the part of professionals to recognise parents' emotional and psychological resources. In *Ended Beginnings: Healing Childbearing Losses* childbirth counsellors Claudia Panuthos and Catherine Romeo stress the need to heed our inner wisdom. 'Are we seeking the best medical care systems or are we looking to be loved by someone in authority?

Do we want to take charge of our lives or would we rather let some-one else, some parent figure, do that for us? The latter choice has robbed far too many childbearing families of the right to birth with-out unneeded intervention and, in some cases, unwanted drugs. Such choices in mental health care can rob us of our long-term psychological health and well-being by shifting the power to heal outside our inner resource system.'

If you have PND you may feel that treatment with drugs is not the answer for you. Mood-altering drugs can remove the symptoms of PND, but can they be said to cure it? Can they actually make matters worse in the long run? Homoeopathic medicine considers treating a disturbance of the system by suppressing the symptoms to be harm-ful, because the symptoms are evidence that the body is attempting to deal with the problem. So it may be that if you feel depressed you do not want prompt 'rescuing', but need to identify with some tragic creative work, such as music or poetry, in order to go deeper into your depression and finally let out the sorrow, misery and pain so that the healing process can then begin. In conventional medicine abscess wounds are kept open until they are completely clean and to encourage healing from the bottom upwards.

Drugs are sometimes given to a woman when it is clear that the socioeconomic circumstances in which she finds herself are over-whelming her, on the basis that it is not possible for any one doctor to change the world so giving drugs to improve the woman's mood and perception of her circumstances is the only help available. But although it is most unlikely that anyone can dramatically improve your circumstances, it is possible to be helped to change your attitude to yourself and your lot so that you can make improvements for yourself. Giving help of this kind can be very time-consuming and is outside the province of most GPs, but doctors or health visitors should be able to indicate where you can find support (see Chapter 6) and means of personal growth (see earlier).

If you are referred for psychotherapy you may feel that the thera-pist is seeing or concentrating on only part of your problem and want to talk to someone else with a more all-embracing approach to your present PND and future mental health. It is worth bearing in mind what is possible in therapy (see Chapter 5) and seeking approaches that promote health and self-actualisation, rather than being only a specific 'cure' for a specific condition, or mechanically readjusting the person to 'normality'.

PND is very prevalent and very real, but is it an illness? Strictly speaking perhaps it is 'a disorder or want of health in mind or body'. And according PND the status of an illness does have the merit of causing the medical profession and society in general to treat PND seriously, appreciate that mothers need help, and consider possible origins and treatments. Yet the connotations of being ill are unfortunate and imply that you cannot really help yourself. 'Being ill' conjures up images of being struck down at random by some malign outside entity, having no say in the matter, being a helpless victim, of requiring expert professional assistance to achieve salvation from the situation.

With so many diseases being brought under control, accepting that you are ill and placing yourself in professional hands carries the expectation that the experts will be able to cure you, and fast. Yet depression is notoriously difficult to treat. It seems more productive to view all forms of PND as manifestations of an organism temporarily thrown out of balance and for women who have PND to join with any professional helpers or lay supporters in looking for ways of slowly recentering themselves.

Many authorities have felt that if PND occurs there must be a reason and that it serves some purpose. That does not mean it should be accepted as inevitable, but that its occurrence should be acknowledged and its significance sought. The NCT's *Pregnancy and Parenthood* says, 'If depression is part of change and growth, perhaps the task is to accept it with information and understanding. By taking away some of the panic and fear of the unknown, inner resources can be mobilised more easily and sharing can take place.'

Too often PND is thought of only in negative terms, as something to be quickly suppressed and banished. But it has its positive sides, too. It is a useful warning that changes are required, within an individual or in their life, and it can result in growth. It might be more helpful in the short-term and avoid future mental disturbances if each individual case of PND were faced by all concerned as something to be lived through and out, while its causes are sought and dealt with, rather than as something that can or should be passively endured or magically cured.

Much of the urge to speedily banish PND arises from the fantasy that we should all be happy, and be seen to be happy, all the time. A permanently painfree state is seen as desirable and normal, and doctors often feel it is their duty to assist everyone to reach and maintain this painfree state, using every scientific weapon in their arsenal. This attitude, on the part of doctor and patient, does not explore the creative and potentially self-healing aspects of suffering, and it certainly does nothing to remove the causes.

The biggest hurdle for anyone with PND who wants to help themselves is accepting that there is actually something fundamentally wrong. You are not just very tired and bad-tempered because the baby wakes you up three times a night, or fed up because you cannot go out dancing any more, or missing your mates at work, or having an off-day (yet again). There is something radically wrong. Things will not get better of their own accord. Something has to change before you break up altogether. The next hurdle, once you realise that you have PND, is being able to walk towards it, explore and evaluate it instead of demanding a (probably unobtainable) quick release. It may be necessary to face up to and embrace a period of instability because it is the prerequisite to change and, without change, there is no development. Change is movement and movement means energy.

We are so fearful of anything unknown that any stirrings and upheavals in our mind and emotions are labelled uncomfortable by us when we first experience them, then abnormal by our circle as they realise something is going on, then pathological by medical authority when it is called on to exorcise the demons. In some cultures the exhibition of disturbance is seen as evidence of being in a spiritual state, 'holy' and in touch with the great life forces. Sadly, this is not so in our culture. But if social pressure forces us to keep on a mask, or if we so fear turmoil that we resist and repress it, we may end up deeply depressed and disturbed. Accepting our manifestations of disturbance and that feeling better will take time allows the work of sorting and mending to go ahead. Being prepared to go down before you come up is vital as it is the acknowledgement of your own pain which provides so much of the power for the healing process (see Chapter 3).

To deal with your PND in a more positive way, try viewing yourself not as the victim of an illness but as the potential survivor of a challenging and enlightening experience.

Considering suicide

Suicidal thoughts are usually kept secret. Even if you are being treated for PND you may feel unable to confide your wish to end it all, to be done with the misery and pain forever. Sometimes the world looks so bleak to mothers that they feel the only answer is to leave it, and to kill their innocent babies to save them from everything. It is rare to find advice for the suicidally depressed. In *Dealing With Depression* Kathy Nairne and Gerrilyn Smith do discuss the desire to die.

'Talking about death is taboo in our society. The idea of choosing to die is even more unacceptable. Wanting to die is therefore the most difficult aspect of depression to talk about. Once again guilt makes it worse. We can feel so guilty at having thought about killing ourselves that we feel even less that we have a right to live, let alone ask for help. If you are thinking about killing yourself and are afraid that you may do it, you must tell someone . . . The suicidal thoughts will lose some of their power when you are able to share them.'

Finding the right person to talk to can be a problem. A friend may refuse to believe you or have to confront their own fears and anxieties before they can help you. A doctor is likely to prescribe medication or consider sending you to stay in a psychiatric ward or hospital. You will usually have to wait to see a psychotherapist or counsellor. Members of self-help groups (see Chapter 6) with informal experience of helping suicidal mothers may be better listeners than close friends, while crisis organisations like the Samaritans (see phone book) or one or the groups that make up the Organisation for Parents Under Stress (see Getting Help) will probably be the most help if you feel desperate.

Nairne and Smith explain that suicidal feelings usually involve ambivalence. 'This means that part of yourself wants to give up and put an end to your life; while another part of you still feels some hope of getting better or some desire to survive and go on struggling. If you can fully acknowledge that part of you that wants to give up, then the more positive side may be able to come through.'

They see some value in having been down to the bottom. 'Feeling suicidal can be a turning point. If you can somehow survive and come through this low point, you may be able to make a real choice to carry on living. You may become more open to change: to living your life on a new basis. You may allow new people into your life, or discover new ideas about what you want for yourself.'

Avoiding depression

There is no guaranteed way of ensuring that you will not get PND but certain steps can improve your physical, mental, emotional and spiritual health before you plan a family and decrease the chances of going downhill in the postnatal period. Some of these measures, which can apply to the way you always look after yourself as well as what you do once you have had a baby, are described earlier in this chapter. This section is concerned with general attitudes to life.

Eliminating negative factors from our lives and introducing practices that are life-enhancing and energising helps to make life less difficult and more joyful, and protects us in times of stress. One negative influence that women often put up with without considering what it is doing to them is continuing in destructive relationships – whether these are with family members, friends or partners. Dealing with tragedies, dramas and stressful events is quite demanding enough. It is asking for trouble to fight a war on two fronts – the enemy at our backs has to be neutralised or go. Oddly enough, we rarely apply the standards of behaviour we expect from strangers to those close to us. Do your nearest and dearest treat you with simple good manners, common kindness and supportive loyalty? If not, and you are a repository for their ill temper and unresolved conflicts while their main purpose seems to undermine you, it is time to have it out with them or say goodbye. If you cannot face ructions and partings, at least keep your distance – minimise meetings and put some emotional space between you.

Some women have no friends but rely completely on their partners and immediate families for social contact. Others have a limited circle of long-established friendships. This complacent and inward-looking attitude is storing up trouble for the future. If your marriage runs into difficulties or your family and old friends move, or you leave work for some time when you have a baby, you can quickly become lonely. Regularly following up opportunities to make new aquaintances and friends will protect you against isolation.

Potential friends do not have to share your every interest or point of view; you do not have to get on with each other's entire families; the friendship can be for a period in your life, not the whole of it. Avoid the habit of shutting people out on the assumption that you can have nothing to say to each other because you come from different cultural or class backgrounds, or another age group. Establishing contact is a two-way process. You cannot blame people for leaving you alone if you keep up a front, put out 'no thank-you' messages or never talk to the people you see around in the street.

Widening your social circle means being more open in your approach, more flexible in your expectations, and less self-protective. You must be willing to risk rejection, on a nothing ventured, nothing gained basis. Because it is more difficult to make this kind of effort when you have just become a mother, and because of the practical ties you will then have, it makes sense to work consciously at building up a circle of aquaintances who like children before you have a baby. This can require a certain amount of organisation if you are out at a job, but it can be done.

Be prepared to offer something of yourself to the community in which you live. For the sake of everyone there, become aware of the local environment and facilities, offering support and campaigning where necessary. The time and energy spent in this way is actually an investment because these things will become of great relevance once you have a child. This generosity will also mean that you are integrated into the community before your baby is born and many more people will take an interest in your welfare when you are pregnant and after the birth, and your baby will be welcomed from the start. Many women also find community work increases their self-confidence enormously.

Forming habits of mind can imply a rigid, unimaginative approach to life. But positive habits can be useful in shaping our outlook and in carrying us through periods of difficulty. The habit of consciously keeping an open mind is not as simple to practise as it seems, but is very valuable. Compartmentalising everything and slamming the lids shut, regarding a particular path as inevitable because you cannot at the moment see a good way out, locks up valuable energy, creates tension and prevents progress being made.

Deliberately leaving things floating loose releases the tension, allows the mind to make connections so that new ideas, insights and solutions arise, apparently of their own accord. Another positive habit to cultivate is being prepared to keep looking at and learning about yourself, and being brave enough to cope with what you learn. The stages of self-discovery – understanding yourself, your feelings and reactions, your needs – are first a vague awareness that something is out of balance and requires looking at, then a gradual formulation of what you find, then communication. All these stages can be disturbing, but the most frightening is the last which requires taking action on the basis of what you have discovered, 'coming out' and saying who you are and what you want of other people. This can sometimes involve disappointing, shocking, angering or alienating people, losing friends or breaking up a relationship. It is a stage through which you may feel your way warily, gradually integrating the new self-knowledge into your life and making it known bit by bit, as and when you feel confident. But it is an important stage of a process that is necessary to ensure constant and healthy growth of an individual's total being.

OPENING YOUR MIND

When you feel your mind closing up, your thoughts beginning to buzz round in ever tightening circles, there is a physical way of breaking out of this negative trap. Sit very comfortably with your back supported and your upturned, open hands resting on your thighs. Let your spine go limp, then your neck and jaw. Let your mouth fall slightly open. Then breathe gently and evenly until the knot of muscle underneath your ribs loosens up. As the blocks in your body vanish, so will the blocks in your mind.

Another practice to follow is trusting our undervalued, much-denigrated intuition. If we can attune ourselves to the messages our intuition sends us we will often find that we already know what is good for us and what will do us harm; what is the way out of our dilemmas, the key to our difficulties.

Some of our experiences can seem at first unpleasant and unnecessary but adopting the view that 'all things are meant' is not mere passive fatalism. Accepting our experiences and seeking to find lessons in them instead of fighting against and rejecting them can bring peace of mind and valuable understanding.

'Life can have the meaning you want it to have' is a more obtainable ideal than 'life can be what you want it to be'. This false formula has led to insatiable and unsatisfiable ambitions that produce relentless pressure and pain, and cause ceaseless and useless struggling against uncontrollable events in our lives. It is also the route to self-pity and defeatism. Some people manage to avoid this while seeing life for what it is. Colin Ward in a *New Society* appraisal of the Russian writer Alexander Herzen speaks of 'his recognition that there are problems for which we will never find solutions, questions to which there are no answers . . . The discovery did not lead him to resignation and inactivity. He did not believe that because no road leads to Utopia, no road leads anywhere.'

Partners in care

Most women who want children prefer to live with a partner and when their relationship runs into a period of stress, which it can after the birth of a child, they feel it is worth persevering with, if only to provide a stable home for their children. This does not necessarily mean they support the mother-as-martyr school, but rather that they have accepted some of the more boring realities of life.

All relationships, not just between partners, require a lot of understanding, give and take and hard work. They go through good and bad patches, change and develop. And it is worth bearing in mind that breakdowns of second marriages run at a higher rate than those of first marriages – getting out may not lead to a better life. Some partners come to accept that they are not particularly close, have a poor sex life or cannot help each other grow. Devotion to their children provides an adequate bond for many couples who believe that you cannot have everything in life, and certainly not all at once.

There is nothing wrong in settling for less than perfection, but not if it involves the woman, the man or both making only male-defined compromises – trying to distort or suppress their needs in order to conform to some ideal of marriage put forward by certain professionals in the field of marriage guidance and psychiatry. Women's perceptions, their priorities, their interpretations of their experiences, their views of what has happened to them or how they would like their relationships and lives to be, must be accepted as valid. This applies to women as professional carers as well as women who are clients.

No woman should put up with obvious or insidious undermining of her self-respect and confidence or verbal abuse, let alone physical violence, from her partner in order to preserve a relationship. To do so is to lay herself open to being gradually destroyed. And if a mother becomes disturbed or depressed postnatally, the marriage hardly seems worth saving if the price is her making all the compromises – especially if she has to be brainwashed, drugged or electrically shocked into acceptance of her situation.

If sorrow or anger about the way her partner treats her and their baby is causing a woman to become depressed, or contributing to depression, it is no good her refusing to acknowledge to herself what is wrong. Holding down these unformulated feelings will cause ill-health – physical or mental. Once a certain stage of awareness is reached, though, there is no going back. It will probably become necessary to confront her partner with her insights and conclusions, to risk a make-or-break outburst of truthfulness. This may make the relationship temporarily worse, but should lead to greater understanding. Whether a couple can then find ways of building bridges and making things work is another matter. Sometimes they may reach an understanding that things cannot ever work, but this is likely to be less damaging for a woman's mental health than suppressing what is troubling her.

There are combinations of expectations and assumptions about parenthood that need to be questioned as they create unnecessary physical and emotional stress for the woman and make their contribution to PND. The main one is that the child is seen as the woman's problem, difficulties with it as things she must get under control lest the child's needs intrude into the couple's relationship. It is somehow her fault if she cannot manage this and her husband feels neglected. It is her fault that there is any problem in the first place.

When there is a specific problem – handicap, hyperactivity, colic, and so on, sometimes a marriage is said to have 'broken down under the strain'. Maybe the pair were not suited anyway, maybe they grew apart during that period when they had no time alone together and parted by mutual agreement. But it often sounds as if the husband could not stand the strain of having a problem child around, and could not cope with his wife having her time and energy fully occupied. The man is then free to walk away from what he does not like coping with – temporarily down to the pub, perhaps eventually out the door for good. The woman is not. She has to cope with her child, and is supposed to try to meet her husband's needs on top of that.

All the time, even if she has actually developed PND, the woman is warned not to exclude her husband, to find time for him, to be alone together. This backed by the implicit blackmail that if a wife expects too much of her husband, is not sufficiently sexually attractive and active, the poor male creature will not be able to survive all the harsh realities, and that there are other women out there who will be only too glad to cosset and cocoon him again.

Mothers need to determinedly ignore this kind of pressure. Much advice aimed at women when they are in dire need of support, reads like a manual on sibling rivalry, not guidance on relationships between consenting adults. Women are frequently advised to treat men in a demeaning way, as children who have not the reserves or maturity or sense to last out through the hard times without constant reassurance and attention. Why are the man's feelings to be so tenderly considered? Life is hard when you grow up, and many women have to grow up, if not overnight, in a very few weeks when their totally dependent child is born. So why cannot the man grow up, too? Why is this too much to expect? Is not the child his as well?

Nowadays, for the majority of couples, having a child is a choice not an accident, and a choice made by both man and woman. Having a child is a serious business. To some extent the party is over. Other hard but rewarding stages of life are to be gone through. Shortage of money and childhood difficulties can make parenthood totally demanding. Then both parents have to work – in or out of the home. So it will be difficult for them to find time for each other. If they both knuckle down and share all tasks and responsibilities they are more likely to have free time together at the end of it all.

All mothers should be able to be confident that their husband supports them or shares the nurturant role, that their children's needs are an unquestioned joint priority. In practice, husbands who share parental and domestic responsibilities are invariably described as 'wonderfully supportive'. What is so wonderful? This is not to knock or belittle what being supportive has cost these men in effort and in overcoming sneering attitudes, and it is usually true that the men who are real sharers do not expect recognition – they just get on with things, feeling it is what they should and want to do. But the question remains. It is clear by the degree of gratitude expressed by women about their partner's helpful behaviour that these men are gems indeed. Why so rare? And why should they be awarded medals for getting on with their responsibilities as partners and parents?

Society currently assumes and accepts that men cannot face parenthood and adulthood in the way women are expected to. The conspiracy that men have more fragile egos needs to be stopped by every mother refusing to be a party to it, expecting more of their partners, and welcoming help when it is offered. In an effort to avoid the stress and misery that results from disparate views about parenthood it is worth discussing expectations in detail before children are born, preferably before a family is planned.

Loving our children

Knowing how to love our children and allowing ourselves to do so is as essential for our mental health and total well-being as it is for theirs. PND itself, or the various stresses that have caused PND, can make it impossible for mothers to feel close to their children, to nurture and enjoy them, and love may only flower properly as depression recedes or circumstances change. But if women allow their views on children to be influenced by the child-hating side of our culture, then the postnatal period is likely to be dominated by negative feelings.

In Britain children are not as valued and integrated into society as they are in many other cultures. They are often viewed as a burden and interference to 'normal' civilised adult life. The birth of a child is assumed to occasion a crisis in the marital relationship, while becoming a mother is held to be a psychological crisis (see later). All these desperately negative points of view condition women to expect motherhood to be difficult and unrewarding and children to bring trouble rather than joy. Some women may concentrate only on the worst aspects of becoming parents and be so confused and resentful that they feel nothing for their newborn babies, or repress their love for them because it is so disturbing.

Professional advice on family relationships invariably reinforces the view that, for a woman, having a man as the centre and mainspring of her life is normal and healthy. The value of other ties, such as with her mother, sisters and friends, is played down. The urge to have children is seen as something to be put in perspective, and involuntary childlessness is seen as a state that it is quite possible for any reasonable female to come to terms with. Putting children before your partner, admitting that they are the most central and vital part of your life, is viewed as obsessional and unhealthy, for mother and child. The possibility that the whole population might end up more emotionally and mentally healthy and that marriages might last longer if parents concentrated more on their children and less on each other is never considered. For this reason those women who are driven by an overwhelming love and tenderness for their babies feel guilty about this, and keep the intensity of their emotions a secret for fear of being thought freaks.

Our society does seem firmly divided into those who love children and those who positively dislike them. Where else in the world would you be told that you are only welcome at social functions and visits to 'friends' if you leave your children behind? Where else would parents be advised they risk spoiling their children if they respond to their needs? Frequently, when a baby cries instead of sleeping, advice is given to first check that nothing obvious is wrong, then to leave the baby to 'cry it out'. This technique needs nerves of steel for the good reason that it is plainly inhumane. It cannot be fair or sensible for desperate babies to be left feeling abandoned when they are incapable of understanding what is going on. Ascribing manipulative tendencies to newborns serves only as an excuse for not being willing or able to meet their needs, and teaches the child that it is alone in the world and cannot trust anyone. Answering babies' needs promptly shows them that you are there for them if needed, and encourages confidence, early independence and psychic wholeness.

The value to both adults and children of parents' giving unconditional love and unconditional positive regard to their babies is little appreciated. Instead, children are reared through a negative system of parental disapproval, based on the withdrawal of love when the child displeases the parent. This system deprives the child and interferes with the way a mother is attuned to her baby. Social worker and writer Elizabeth Hormann, in the American *Mothering*, emphasises the value of being in touch with and responsive to your baby. 'Children who are, from birth on, in close physical contact with other people are most likely to have their physical and emotional needs met. Ideally (though there are other ways to accomplish it) this means breastfeeding and unrestricted access to at least one parent. Sharing a bed and bath, hugging, kissing and gentle rough-housing are all ways parents get in touch with their children.' A baby whose needs are met is likely to be easier to deal with and more rewarding than one who feels short-changed from birth.

Perhaps those who fail to respond to babies' messages and treat them with indifference, lack of understanding or downright cruelty do so because they do not regard babies as real people. Clinical and research psychologist Valerie Yule reports in *New Society* that she heard the young parents of a six-week-old baby say proudly, 'We know other parents who smack their babies to keep them quiet. We think that is terrible. All you need to do is shake them.' In her own research study of the behaviour of parents and children in public she observed indifference, brusqueness, intolerance and smacks. She ends her article, 'Some people are involved in arguments about when an embryo becomes human. This is an urgent question today, but it has a strange quality about it when young parents ask you in all seriousness, "When does a child become human?" '

Britain has a high level of recorded incidences of child abuse – concerned agencies are faced with a flood of cases of violence, torture, starvation and sexual molestation. 'Why is it happening? Don't we love our children?' asks Liz Hodgkinson in the *Sunday Mirror*. According to child expert David Pithers whom she interviewed, the answer is an empahatic no. He believes that, as a nation, we actually hate small children. Mr Pithers, a psychotherapist with the National Children's Home, says, 'When our children cry we hit them.'

He blames the dramatic rise in child abuse cases in part on immaturity. 'People do not grow up themselves before they start a family. They can't cope and they lash out at the nearest available object – the child.' And he believes many people have children for the wrong reasons. 'Those who have little love in their lives have children because they want to be loved by them . . . Immature parents are quickly disappointed by their children who are not loving but who scream, make demands and are a continual nuisance.'

In a woman who has not yet reached a certain level of maturity, or made good her own early deprivations, the unremitting needs of a dependent newborn can induce total panic – she may feel she is being consumed by her baby's demands. To stop these feelings she will either react against the baby, maybe with violence, or cut off from responding to it at all.

If other people's babies make you feel helpless, inadequate or angry when they cry it may be necessary to think very carefully about how far you have to develop before you are ready to have children. It is true that it is easier to know what is wrong with your own baby and to be able to do something to put things right. Against that, though, is the fact that you cannot walk away, handing your baby to someone else. The various stresses of motherhood could combine to either make a bad relationship between you and your baby, or to make you depressed and disturbed, or both.

270

Parenthood, particularly motherhood, is hard work, but so are all rewarding projects. It is helpful to be warned that babies are not little cherubs; they need endless attention and cry long and loud when they do not get it. But expectations govern perceptions. If all you read and hear about and therefore concentrate on, is what boring, monotonous drudgery motherhood is you could end up resenting everything you do for your dependent baby and wishing away the first months and years of its life instead of relishing every fast-vanishing moment.

Fortunately, it is possible to find other more positive and encouraging views about caring for children. Some parents see the hours spent with our babies as a unique opportunity, allowing us, even forcing us, to slow down enough to develop a different perspective on life. Observing and interacting with our babies, allowing ourselves to be acutely in touch with them, can bring enormous pleasure, add new dimensions, bring fresh insights, and seem like a second chance in one's own life.

In a Handy Hints leaflet, under the heading It's Not Forever, the ABM say, 'Remember that despite the amount of time it takes to care for and feed a young baby, they are fun, as every day brings new developments from the first smile to the first tooth to the first step. If you can really enjoy this precious time with your baby the hard work becomes very worthwhile.'

It is so unusual to take open, obvious pleasure in our babies that we almost need permission for this indulgence. In Canada's *Compleat Mother* Sheila Stubbs says, 'The smartest thing I ever did was to go to a La Leche League meeting . . . What I found was a group of mothers who actually *enjoyed* their babies. They didn't look at their situation as if it was just one of the rotten parts about life that you hurry and get over with so you can get back to normal, which we see so prominent today . . . I was impressed by the fact that they simply reassured me that I was doing the right thing trusting my instincts, and picking the baby up every time he cried. After all, nobody was ever spoiled by love. I kept going back to the meetings, hungry for more information, and kept learning the secrets of enjoying my baby, just by observing . . . Best of all I found a style of mothering, far easier than most. LLL teaches not just a method of feeding, but a style that makes motherhood truly a joy.'

The more you know about the early development of babies, in the womb – and evidence is being accumulated of how much the child's awareness is functioning from the earliest weeks after conception –

and during the early weeks after birth, the more you will regard your baby as a small person with messages to communicate to you and lessons to teach you. Willingness to learn the baby's language can turn the postnatal period into one of fascinating and rewarding exploration, instead of seeing it as merely marking time or an exercise in bare survival.

One of the principles on which Maria Montessori's life work on education and child development was based was that of being guided by the child and open to him. In *The Secret of Childhood* she spoke of 'discovering the child' in order to effect his liberation. She believed that 'Behind every surprising response on the part of the child lies an enigma to be deciphered,' and said that adults should examine themselves methodically to discover defects that could become obstacles in their relations with children. To her the worst obstacles, 'the deadliest sins', were anger and pride which fused together to assume the form of tyranny, subduing and opressing the child's spirit. She recommended that adults strip themselves of pride and anger, become humble and charitable. She said, 'there must be a radical change in our inner state, which prevents us as adults from understanding [children].'

Maria Montessori said that children want to love adults, delight in being with them, yet 'The adult passes by this mystical love without perceiving it. But the little one who so loves us will grow up, will vanish. And who will ever love us as he does? . . . We defend ourselves against this love that will pass away, and we shall never find anything to equal it. We in our turmoil say, "I haven't time, I can't, I have a lot to do," and we think in our hearts, "The child must be taught better, or he will make us his slaves." What we want is to be free of him to do what we ourselves like doing, so as not to give up our convenience.'

So, what are our babies trying to tell us, and what can we learn from close contact? The more we can see their point of view, the more reasonable their behaviour seems. For example, writing in *Mothering* on coping with your baby's crying, Sandy Jones says, 'Our grandmothers used to claim that some babies cry simply because they don't like being here. Knowing how violent birth is for many babies and how most of us have forgotten the primitive human language of transferring energy to our babies rather than simply talking to them, gives plausibility to the idea that very precocious, bright babies may have a deep sense of grief and protest at their very existence.'

Other parents writing in *Mothering* have seen positive merit in the seclusion, isolation and narrow focusing that the early weeks to some extent enforce. Lay midwife Nan Koehler feels that it is a good thing to stay at home exclusively with a tiny baby in a quiet environment as this allows time for mother and baby to become attuned to each other. 'Bonding can only occur as the result of days on end of mindless routine and the total attention of the mother on the child . . . The biological results of this isolation are a tranquil child and an intense telepathic relationship between mother and child.' This period of exclusivity is only possible with the support of other experienced mothers. 'In order to stay home we must allow other women into our home.' She even sees a place in our development for lack of sleep. 'People pay money to go to retreats where they can't sleep and must fast to enter the state that all nursing mothers are in who really take loving care of their babies. The combination of sleep deprivation and constant selfless service, taken in stride with grace and humour, prepare the woman for any challenge in later life.'

This idea of the value of night waking is echoed by another parent in the same magazine. 'Sleep deprivation and the intensity of the first weeks combine to induce a definite altered state of consciousness,' says Victor La Cerva. Describing himself as a paediatrician and child at heart, he sets out his views of what children can give us, if we let them, in a Dearest Papa 'letter' to him from his newborn daughter.

'I can teach you to be in the present, which will allow you to become more conscious and aware . . . Because I view the world through the eyes of the present, there is always so much that is new. Do you not see some lessons for your own life in me? I am your unconscious connection as well. I am closer to that collective flow of humanity that is unspoken yet very much felt . . . I can also put you in touch with your unconscious through my night wakings, multiple opportunities for remembering your dreams . . . And, of course, I constantly trigger your emotional life, serving as a mirror within which you can see your deepest self, if you are willing to look . . . I test the limits of your patience, releasing your anger at times and giving you more opportunities for increased self-awareness . . .

'So, I offer you pure experience, lots of practice in being in the present, a taste of communication with the unconscious, and constant insight into your emotional life; along with much joy and laughter to fill your days and nights. As I emerge from the safety of the womb, I invite you to transcend the boundaries of your self-awareness. I hope that you will reflect and act upon the ideas I have shared in this letter. Remember that ideas, over time, have a way of attaining biological reality. Surrender to the flow of life that I represent. When you are with me, be conscious of your thoughts and actions, for they will provide the feedback you need for growth. Relax, enjoy and trust your feelings and intuitions. Life provides, for both of us.'

Motherhood: a happy progression

While pregnancy, birth and the postnatal months are certainly a period of adjustment, the view of some professionals in the mental health care and counselling fields that parenthood equals problems seems overly pessimistic. The Thomas Coram Research Unit found that one year after the birth 37% of mothers and 51% of fathers in a study rated having a child as improving their marriage as against 21% and 15% who said the child worsened the marriage or they had a mixed reaction.

'Crisis' has different connotations for different people – neutral, negative or positive. When describing the birth of a child as causing a crisis in the marital relationship, or motherhood as a maturational crisis, professionals tend to look at these as occasions when things are likely to go awry and their views filter through to mothers who may interpret any changes as inevitably for the worst. Fortunately, more optimistic views exist. The authors of one study on pregnancy and the postnatal period (Shereshefsky and Yarrow 1974) concluded that 'in the use of the term crisis in the sense of a transitional phase or its dictionary definition of a "turning point", our young women and their husbands were indeed involved in a crisis.' But, 'If the term "pregnancy-as-crisis" is used to mean a stress involving threat or loss and requiring resources beyond the ordinary, then our data suggest that a first pregnancy is not, generally, a crisis in these terms.' They also saw another dimension. 'Pregnancy was also a turning point in terms of inner reality in that it allowed or even forced the woman to become aware of her intrapsychic self – of her body image and her feeling responses especially. The impact on the man's self-concepts was often of equal force.'

In examining the period of pregnancy and after, Dr Elliott reports that psychoanalyst and author Dana Breen (in a 1975 study) employs 'a positive developmental view of pregnancy and "delivery" as opposed to the negative, temporary disequilibrium model of the "crisis" viewpoint. She portrays this as a "stage" in development, part of maturation, rather than as a hurdle with a potential for unstable change. Her study was designed to demonstrate this development and to show that "the healthy woman is the one who can modify her perception of herself and her relationship with members of her family in a way congruent with the new situation of having a child".'

Many authorities believe that a healthy emotional and mental outcome of pregnancy consists of a return to the woman's pre-pregnancy state after a period of disequilibrium, and much advice to new mothers generally and those with PND in particular emphasises 'getting back to normal'. Any woman who is made to feel that she should be aiming at a return to her pre-pregnancy state is being mislead into trying to achieve what is both impossible and undesirable. There is no going back.

Misunderstandings by professionals and mothers of the period of change following birth can cause problems in several ways. The assumption that birth precipitates an emotional crisis diverts attention from the possibility that there are recitifiable physical causes for unusual behaviour. Attempts can be made to reduce extreme exhaustion and remedy biochemical imbalances, both of which result in mood changes. The mother's 'loss' of her old persona may occasion sadness and mourning which, if she recognises it for what it is, will be self-limiting. But her reactions may be misinterpreted as endogenous clinical depression, requiring treatment with drugs. In fact, whenever women start reacting to stressful situations, or exhibiting signs of the upheaval going on in their heads and hearts, their behaviour is likely to be categorised as abnormal and requiring treatment.

Holding to the ideal of a return to normality, and striving to realise the expectation, is stressful and damaging to mothers. The attempt leads them up false avenues and ignores the growth potential of the birth experience and the maturational processes that becoming a mother involves. Mothers may use up precious energy and become ill, resisting change instead of opening themselves to the positive aspects of what is happening to them, seeing themselves as different and potentially more complete. Advice to go back to the pre-pregnancy emotional and psychological state, and to curb the fluctuation of emotions following birth, is advice to throw away a unique chance to develop and may cause or increase disturbance and depression.

Caring for a newborn baby, and birth itself, provide chances to become wiser and stronger, to get back in touch with ourselves and with the primal life force. Taking yourself through the birth experience, rather than wondering what hit you or handing yourself over body and soul to the experts, is a character-forming experience. It is considered admirable to undertake challenging physical feats or geographical journeys, but bizarre and unhealthily masochistic to approach birth with the same sense of excitement and hope of feeling triumphant.

If you have what, in your own terms, is 'a good birth' you will grow through that, very dramatically because it is such a momentous event. You will be stronger and trust yourself more. Routine interventions rob you of this opportunity for growth, deny you the fullness of this challenging experience, undermine your trust in yourself and your body to see you through, distract you from your effort, absorption and abandonment. They also interfere with hormonal output. It is clearly important for your emotional, mental and physical well-being to avoid interventions wherever possible.

Women feel powerfully drawn to the experience of birth itself, as opposed to just wanting children and knowing that desire necessitates enduring birth. One mother of four, quoted by Dr Dick-Read, said 'I look forward to the conflict with my body, the struggle with my mind and the certainty of that glorious finale. It is a wonderful experience that I must repeat again and again – I feel that with each child I am a better mother to them all.'

To Dr Dick-Read birth called on a lot of qualities and could have rich rewards for women's whole personalities. He felt that birth had a unique role to play. 'It is the greatest experience of a woman's life and can establish her emotional control and self-confidence for all time.' And he said 'Many women realise that the birth of their child altered their whole attitude to life. It seemed that until then they had been waiting for something without which they were immature and imperfect; they did not realise that it was motherhood till the postnatal revelation opened their eyes.'

If you treat birth as a project for which you need to prepare yourself physically, mentally, emotionally and spiritually it is likely to go well and be much more rewarding. Birth is a challenge. The challenge is not to do it 'right' or 'successfully' or better than other mothers. The challenge is to grow through using the aspects of your character called on during birth.

Facing birth does require guts. Not, as usually assumed, to deal with

276

the pain (which for many women is perfectly bearable and for a few scarcely exists). The question is, will you have the guts to abandon yourself utterly and *let* the birth happen? Will you be able to allow your intuition to guide you when to control yourself and when to let go? Birth involves struggle, too. It is not the commonly perceived struggle against the body to get the baby out, but an effort to become exactly in tune with your body, to let it work perfectly by itself, without impeding it, the struggle to stop interfering and let it be.

The real challenge of birth is that you can only do it yourself. You can be coached and led, then accompanied, but you give birth alone. Facing up to that thrilling, awesome prospect allows the actual birth to be followed by an enormous sense of attainment and triumph, waves of energy and power, and a tremendous 'high'.

Because of the present tendency of our society to control birth, to attempt to get through it with minimum impact, to refuse to discuss the experience or the feelings it arouses, to get it over and done with, out of the way and everything back to normal as fast as possible, women often do not get a chance to acknowledge and work through their feelings and reactions, communicate them, or establish that they are common. Many mothers fear that their extremes of feeling at the birth and afterwards are a sign of derangement, so they keep what is going on secret or even refuse to acknowledge it to themselves. The emotions that arise in women during and after birth range from power to panic. Exhibiting them may result in being labelled psychotic, manic, depressed, wierd or inadequate. Suppressing the emotions, feeling guilty about them, worrying that you are going mad, can result in actual depression or disturbance.

One little-acknowledged feeling is the tremendous power a mother feels within herself, having given birth. This sense of power may be totally unexpected and profoundly disconcerting to her. And, judging by the many birth procedures which strip mothers of their authority and render them powerless, it is, if only subconsciously so, disconcerting to non-mothers, female as well as male.

In her book *The Mother Knot* Jane Lazarre describes her own coming to terms with the knowledge of this power after the difficult birth of her first baby. 'As I wandered my way through long, solitary days, in that apparent inactivity, I was courting and accepting the truth I had been trying to deny.' There was something 'which had to do with a part of myself which was always frustrating me by remaining hidden despite my conscious attempts to express it. It kept hidden because it

277

was frightened, frightened of its own power . . . Pregnancy and child-birth had exposed that power, made it impossible for me to ever deny it again. There it was: I had created a child . . . I was obsessed with that excruciating, uncivilised, powerful moment of birth, imprisoned like a Van Gogh in a frame in the sterile white and green delivery room which was dotted by the fatigued faces of the nurses and doctors who wanted to get home to bed. I was in the grip of a loving fascination with my own power.'

Another emotion whose strength can stun and disturb mothers is the fierce love they feel for their newborns plus the accompanying ruthless urge to protect them. Many women face in secret and for the first time the sure knowledge that they could kill anyone, even their previously nearest and dearest, if they had to save their baby. In a world where the need for such drastic action does not arise having these thoughts may seem monstrous, sick and wicked. But it is more unhealthy to hide from the strength of our instincts.

At the other end of the spectrum from feelings of protectiveness and power is panic at the realisation that your baby is real and here to stay. This is it, you are a mother. Along with the awareness of total responsibility there comes a heartbreaking sense of your baby's fragility, innocence and trust. By comparison the world into which it has been born seems unutterably bleak, meaninglessly destructive, indiscriminately cruel, terrifyingly dangerous and hostile. It is easy to feel overwhelmed by the idea that, in the face of all this, you will be helpless to protect your child. If you are unhappy with the way your partner disregards your feelings, or you had a birth in which other people's wishes were imposed on you, your sense of powerlessness may be compounded – 'If I cannot protect myself, how can I protect my baby?' Mothers who are unprotected and unsupported are particularly vulnerable to an acute crisis of confidence in themselves, and an agonising awareness of just how alone they are and what odds they must face.

It is generally accepted that the biochemical changes and hormonal adjustments following birth, which need not cause feelings of depression or dramatic mood changes but which commonly do so because they are disrupted by other factors, are the main element contributing to the postnatal blues. But, in addition, feeling powerless to protect your baby, whether from a nuclear holocaust or from unnecessary postnatal medical procedures, is profoundly disturbing and depressing. The weepiness that is so little understood and so lightly dismissed may be tears of fear and anger. In turn, these emotions can interfere with smooth biochemical readjustment, creating further distressing mood changes. Mothers who had a good and gentle birth, who feel thankful and strong, may weep with the utter joy of how wonderful it is to give birth. Those tears, too, may be misconstrued and hurried away. It is assumed that the mother is on a near-manic high from which she will descend with an awful crash into deep, maybe psychotic depression.

Women are categorised as 'emotionally labile' after birth, as if flowing this way and that is a bad state of affairs to be got over as soon as possible. Some of their extremes of mood and depression are probably attributable to undesirable negative factors over which they have little or no control but which could be changed if we all felt it was worthwhile for birth and motherhood to be happier. But some fluctuations in mood, that are misunderstood and disapproved of, represent a reawakening of blunted sensibilities. To survive, most of us learn from earliest childhood not to feel to the fullest, not to respond, not to react. Pregnancy and birth, the presence of a tiny creature who is all feeling and responds uninhibitedly and fully to every sensation, restores in some degree our true level of sensitivity. But in a cruel world, the shock and pain of so much feeling, of such heightened awareness, can be too much. As intense feelings come back, so it is necessary to give them expression – laughing one moment, crying in joy or agony the next. This is not 'being ill'. This is being fully human.

Mothers need time after the birth to register and understand the array of new emotions they feel. It helps to know in advance that your emotions may be bewildering in their variety and overwhelming in their intensity and that this is not 'abnormal'. Motherhood is less likely to result in emotional and mental disturbance if we are willing to welcome and be carried along by the feelings that are aroused. The nature of birth means surrendering control and we must learn not to fear this. A flood of powerful feelings will be unleashed by birth and being a mother and we need to know that it is all right, it is a sign of health not sickness, to let go. If we can open ourselves to giving birth and to what we feel, motherhood will be a happier experience.

279

Conclusion

We are physical, mental, emotional and spiritual beings and where any dysfunction occurs, even if it is obvious in one area only, the whole organism must be considered. I believe this is true of emotional and mental disturbances postnatally and that there can be no single, narrow definition of PND, one simple cause, one solution. PND is itself a symptom that something deeper and more complicated is amiss. Finding quite what this is in any individual woman requires an open mind and creative imagination, but I think the way in which all three forms of PND happen follows a basic pattern.

Pregnancy and birth produce biochemical changes to which women's bodies are able to adapt. The period following birth is one of further changes and adaptation, which it should be normal to pass through smoothly. If however, a mother is stressed to an unusual degree in her life generally or around the time of the birth, for one or a mixture of reasons, biochemical readjustment will be disrupted, resulting in alterations in brain chemistry that produce changes and disturbances, such as anxiety, depression and mania.

So, in some women the symptoms of PND are caused by the action of stresses on the biochemical system around the time of birth countering the body's usual ability to restore its balance after birth. Alternatively, where the biochemical system is already somewhat out of balance before pregnancy starts, due to inherited factors or earlier stresses from various sources, the dramatic biochemical changes produced by birth may be more than these handicapped systems can deal with. The difficulties will be further compounded if these women experience additional stresses around the time of birth.

A woman may be chronically stressed before becoming a mother by reason of:

- unresolved psychological conflicts
- problematic present relationships
- adverse socioeconomic circumstances
- nutritional deficiencies and imbalances
- environmental chemicals

Alternatively, or additionally, she may be stressed during and after birth by reason of:

- the type of birth she experiences
- the stirring up, by birth and motherhood, of long-hidden emotional conflicts
- problems in adjusting to motherhood
- her partner's difficulties in adjusting to fatherhood
- lack of emotional or practical support
- worsened socioeconomic circumstances
- freshly created nutritional deficiencies and imbalances
- the continued presence of environmental chemicals

The term PND is misused in certain cases. Some of what is labelled postnatal mental illness should be described as 'postnatal distress': a woman may be deeply unhappy or angry rather than disturbed. Other supposed cases of PND may not even be postnatal distress, merely evidence that a woman is working through important emotional changes. Certain women who become depressed postnatally, if they keep a careful diary of their symptoms, may find these are cyclical and that they have PMS not PND.

I have emphasised the role of nutrition and allergies in PND. This field is controversial and under-researched but, I think, will be found to have critical relevance to the well-being of new mothers. Of course, careful nutrition plus the detection of allergies should not be looked to in isolation to prevent or remove PND; total stress load needs to be considered as well. However stress, and the deeper damage it has done, cannot always be avoided or removed quickly, and good nutrition does serve an invaluable role in protecting and strengthening the body's resistance.

Believing that biochemical imbalances are the immediate cause of the symptom of PND does not imply any acceptance on my part that these imbalances are inevitable (or untreatable). Women's bodies are

281

tough, complicated and highly adaptive, as they need to be to produce and nurture healthy children. So there is no 'natural' inherent reason why such a proportion of women should succumb to PND.

The steady rate of incidence, geographically and historically, is often cited as evidence that PND is 'normal'. But it is more likely to be evidence that, universally, women have to battle against greater stresses than men, and that too often they reach childbirth and motherhood in an unnecessarily weakened state. Psychological stresses can affect any individual, regardless of gender or class. Other adverse circumstances affect both sexes of whole classes – poverty, poor housing, harsh working conditions. But within most societies women get a raw deal in terms of the value set on them and their needs, the amount of grinding, unremitting work they do, the quantity and quality of food they get, personal freedom and choice, and opportunities to receive emotional support and spiritual nourishment. They are also supposed to absorb the results of the stress their husbands and children experience outside the home.

Most of the stresses have socioeconomic causes and are open to political solutions. Mothers who get PND do not do so because their biochemistry goes haywire as a result of giving birth. They get PND because their highly stressed systems are fighting a losing battle after birth. Decreasing the sources of stress is a matter of personal and public will. We could change society, and make the way women experience birth and motherhood happier . . . *if* we all wanted to.

Appendix

GETTING HELP

Like the rest of this book, Getting Help is intended for women who have postnatal depression or wish to try to avoid it; for mothers who are distressed or angry postnatally; for partners, family and friends; or for anyone who is giving thought to the whole business of having children. The publications listed are a small selection of books (mostly paperbacks) and booklets that are helpful or thought-provoking, plus some directories of therapists, counsellors, voluntary organisations and self-help groups. Many of the publications contain reading lists and contacts for helpful organisations.

The organisations mentioned here provide support and factual information; some are also involved in campaigning work. Most offer resource lists of local branches and like-minded groups to contact, plus lists of their own publications or recommended reading, and new publications are reviewed in their newsletters. For reasons of space it has not been possible to give more than one contact for each organisation who will supply details of help nationwide.

The addresses and telephone numbers of organisations are correct at the time of going to press but, as many are run on a voluntary basis or depend on uncertain funding, it is possible they will change. Please send a large sae (250 × 176mm) with all enquiries to the groups listed.

Chapter 1

Suggested reading

Motherhood and Mental Illness ed I F Brockington and R Kumar (Academic Press, 1982, £25)

Postnatal Depression: A Guide for Health Professionals John L Cox (Churchill Livingstone, 1986)

Mental Illness in Pregnancy and the Puerperium ed M Sandler (Oxford University Press, 1978, £25)

Chapter 2

Suggested reading

Naturebirth: Preparing for Joyful Birth in an Age of Technology Danaë Brook (Penguin, 1986)

Childbirth Without Fear: The Original Approach to Natural Childbirth Grantly Dick-Read MD; revised and edited by Helen Wessel and Harlan F Ellis MD (Harper & Row, 1985)

Birthrights: A Parents' Guide to Modern Childbirth Sally Inch (Hutchinson, 1982)

The Experience of Childbirth Sheila Kitzinger (Gollanz, 1962); plus other books and publications

Pregnancy and Childbirth: Your Right to Have It Your Own Way Nicky Wesson (Thorsons, 1987)

Maternity Care in Action: A Guide to Good Practice and a Plan for Action. Reports from the Maternity Services Advisory Committee (HMSO). Part 1 – Antenatal Care, 1982 (55p); Part 2 – Care During Childbirth, 1984 (75p); Part 3 – Care of the Mother and Baby, 1985 (95p)

Helpful organisations

NCT

(National Childbirth Trust)
9 Queensborough Terrace
London W2 3TB
(01–221 3833)

AIMS

(Association for Improvements in the Maternity Services)
Hon Secretary
163 Liverpool Road
London N1 ORF

Maternity Alliance

59–61 Camden High Street
London NW1 7JL
(01–388 6337)

Dick-Read School for Natural Birth

Mrs Prunella Briance
14 Pitt Street
London W8
(01–937 4140)

Society to Support Home Confinement

Margaret Whyte
Lydgate House
Lydgate Lane
Wolsingham
Co Durham DL13 3HA
(0388 528044)

Chapter 3

Suggested reading

The Essential Father Tony Bradman (Unwin, 1983)

Talking with Mothers Dana Breen (Jill Norman, 1981); plus other books

Women Confined: Towards a Sociology of Childbirth Ann Oakley (Martin Robertson, 1980); plus other books and publications

Women and the Psychiatric Paradox P Susan Penfold and Gillian A Walker (Open University Press, 1984)

The Uncertain Father Richard Seel (Gateway Books, 1987)

The Superwoman Syndrome Marjorie Shaevitz (Fontana, 1985)

Round About Fifty Hours a Week: The Time Costs of Children David Piachaud (CPAG, £1.75 inc p&p)

Becoming a Father (NCT, 25p)

Helpful organisations

Marriage Guidance Councils

see phone books, libraries, clinics, local newspapers

Women's Aid Federation England

(c/o 01–251 6537)

Incest Crisis Line

(01–890 4732 or 01–422 5100)

Rape crisis centres

see phone books, or Spare Rib *publish a nationwide list each month*

National Childcare Campaign

Wesley House
70 Great Queen Street
London WC2B 5AX
(01–405 5617)

National Council for One Parent Families

255 Kentish Town Road
London NW5 2LX
(01–267 1361)

CPAG

(Child Poverty Action Group)
1 Macklin Street
London WC2B 5NH
(01–242 3225)

Women's Reproductive Rights Information Centre

52–54 Featherstone Street
London EC1
(01–251 6332)

Chapter 4

Suggested reading

The Zinc Solution Prof Derek Bryce-Smith and Liz Hodgkinson (Century Arrow, 1986)

Candida Albicans Leon Chaitow (Thorsons, 1985)

Depression After Childbirth: How to Recognize and Treat Postnatal Illness Katharina Dalton (Oxford University Press, 1980); plus other books

The Bitter Pill Dr Ellen Grant (Corgi, 1986)

The Pill Dr John Guillebaud (Oxford University Press, 1984)

Not All in the Mind Dr Richard Mackarness (Pan, 1976)

Allergies: What Everyone Should Know Keith Mumby MB, ChB (Unwin, 1986)

Zinc and Other Micro-Nutrients Dr Carl C Pfeiffer (Pivot, USA, 1978)

The Premenstrual Syndrome: The Curse That Can Be Cured Dr Caroline Shreeve (Thorsons, 1983)

Nutrition Against Disease Dr Roger J Williams (Bantam, 1973)

Anxiety, Depression and Nutrition Dr Barrie R Bartlett (Larkhall Laboratories, 45p inc p&p)

Understanding Allergies Ellen Rothera (Food and Chemical Allergy Association, £1 + 13p p&p)

Helpful organisations

Foresight

(The Association for the Promotion of Preconceptual Care)
Mrs Peter Barnes
The Old Vicarage
Church Lane
Witley
Godalming
Surrey GU8 5PN

send sae for name of nearest clinician

Institute for Optimum Nutrition

5 Jerdan Place
London SW6 1BE
(01–385 7984/8673)

Action Against Allergy

43 The Downs
London SW20 8HG
(01–947 5082)

Food and Chemical Allergy Association

27 Ferringham Lane
Ferring
West Sussex
(0903 41178)

NSRA

(National Society for Research into Allergy)
PO Box 45
Hinckley
Leicestershire LE10 1JY
(0455 635212)

PMT Advisory Service

PO Box 268
Hove
East Sussex BN3 1RW
(0273 771366)

Miscellaneous

Progesterone treatment Dr Dalton will supply details to women who cannot get information through their GP or antenatal clinic and to professionals who look after pregnant women and new mothers. 100 Harley Street, London W1A 4AE (01-935 2146)

Zinc levels Nature's Best supply Zincatest, a low-cost combined 'taste test' for assessing zinc levels and zinc supplement.

Evening primrose oil Several companies, including Efamol, offer EPO supplements. Some people find these difficult to tolerate digestively. Larkhall Laboratories sell FF-100 dry tablets which are easier to digest and absorb, so reducing the quantity necessary to take.

Mail order Larkhall Laboratories offer services, information and a wide range of health products. They publish a newsletter and large fact-packed catalogue which includes a book list. 225 Putney Bridge Road, London SW15 2PY (01–870 0971).
Nature's Best offer information, advice and a wide range of health products. They publish a full catalogue which includes a book list and details of over 100 newsletters on nutritional and related subjects (15p each). PO Box 1, 1 Lamberts Road, Tunbridge Wells TN2 3EQ (0892 34143).
Wholefood publish an extensive booklist which includes American, rare and out of print books. Send large sae to 24 Paddington Street, London W1M 4DR (01-935 3924).

Directory of Allergy Societies and Other Organisations (NSRA, 50p inc p&p)

Tracing allergies Larkhall Laboratories provide Cytotoxic blood testing for masked food allergies. Panels A, B and C cover main groups of goods. One panel, £30; two panels, £55; three panels, £80 (including computerised diet).
Biolab Medical Unit provide a blood, sweat and hair test for £55. The Stone House, 9 Weymouth Street, London WLN 3FF (01-636 5959).

Pure water The general public have the right to request full analytical details of their water supply at source by a phone call or letter to the Customer and Data Services Department of their water board. If a householder wants their tap water analysed the water board may do this for a charge or refer them to a local public analyst.
The Brita water filter jug (£10) is available from health and department stores. Brita (UK) Ltd, Ashley Road, Walton on Thames, Surrey KT12 1HG.

Chapter 5

Suggested reading

Understanding Mental Health Angelina Gibbs (Which? Books, 1986)

A Complete Guide to Therapy Joel Kovel (Pelican)

The Mind Benders: The Use of Drugs in Psychiatry Prof Malcolm Lader (MIND Bookshop, 155 Woodhouse Lane, Leeds 2; £1.15 inc p&p)

Helpful organisations

MIND

(The National Association for Mental Health)
22 Harley Street
London W1N 2ED
(01–637 0741)

Women's Therapy Centre

6 Manor Gardens
London N7
(01–263 6200)

Samaritans

24-hour service for anyone in distress or suicidal, see phone books

Miscellaneous

MIND publish reading and resource lists. They do not provide psychotherapy or counselling services, but do keep a list of institutions and organisations which offer psychotherapy. Send large sae marked Psychotherapy List to the Information Unit. MIND's regional resource centres have information on opportunities for psychotherapy outside London.

The British Association for Counselling (0788 78328) publish an annually revised *Counselling Resources Directory* (£12.50).

Chapter 6

Suggested reading

How to Survive as a Working Mother Lesley Garner (Penguin, 1982)

Crying Baby: How to Cope Pat Gray (Wisebuy Publications, PO Box 379, London NW3 1NJ; £3.50 + 40p p&p)

Encourage the Mother Peggy Thomas (ABM, £2 + 25p p&p)

Mothers Writing About Postnatal Depression (NCT, 80p + 20p p&p)

Mothers Writing About the Death of a Baby (NCT, £1 + 20p p&p)

The Emotions and Experiences of Some Disabled Mothers (NCT, £1 + 20p p&p)

You Are Not Alone (Depressives Associated, 50p + 13p p&p)

Trouble With Tranquillisers (Release, 50p inc p&p)

Helpful Organisations

Local information Libaries, ethnic centres, places of worship, doctors' surgeries, child health clinics, health visitors and social services departments of local councils all have details of local organisations, such as women's centres, PND support groups (if any), postnatal support groups, mother and baby/toddler schemes, playgroups, groups for single parents, disabled parents, and parents of children with handicaps and genetic diseases. Libraries stock some directories and should be able to supply national addresses of relevant organisations.

Association for Post-Natal Illness

7 Gowan Avenue
London SW6 6RH

NCT see Chapter 2

Sheffied Post-Natal Depression Support Group

Agnes Burns
4 High Hazels Mead
Handsworth
Sheffield S9 4NU

Depressives Associated

PO Box 5
Castletown
Portland
Dorset DT5 1BQ

Pacific Post Partum Support Society

888 Burrard Street
Vancouver
BC V6Z 1X9
Canada

ABM

(Association of Breastfeeding Mothers)
131 Mayow Road
London SE26
(01–778 4769)

LLL

(La Leche League)
BM 3424
London WC1V 6XX
(01–404 5011)

Working Mothers Association

7 Spencer Walk
London SW15 1PL
(01–788 2565)

Disabled Living Foundation

380–384 Harrow Road
London W9 2HU
(01–289 6111)

Cry-sis

BM Cry-sis
London WC1N 3XX
(01–404 5011)

HCSG

(Hyperactive Children's Support Group)
71 Whyke Lane
Chichester
West Sussex PO19 2LD

Caesarian Support Group of Cambridge

Katherine Steele
7 Aylestone Road
Cambridge CB4 1HF

NIPPERS

(National Information for Parents of Prematures: Education Resources and Support)
c/o Sam Segal
Perinatal Unit
St Mary's Hospital
Praed Street
London W2 1NY

The Miscarriage Association

18 Stoneybrook Close
West Bretton
Wakefield WF4 4TP
(092 485 515)

SANDS

(Stillbirth and Neonatal Death Society)
Argyle House
29–31 Euston Road
London NW1 2SD
(01–833 2851)

NSPCC

(National Society for the Prevention of Cruelty to Children)
67 Saffron Hill
London EC1N 8RS
(01–242 1626 *and phone books)*

Home-Start Consultancy

140 New Walk
Leicester LE1 7JL
(0533 554988)

OPUS

(Organisations for Parents Under Stress)
106 Godstone Road
Whyteleafe CR3 OEB
(01–645 0469)

Release

(c/o 01–603 8654)
information on drugs

Alcoholics Anonymous

PO Box 514
11 Redcliffe Gardens
London SW10 9BG
(01–352 9799 *and phone books*)

MAMA

(Meet-a-Mum Association)
Kate Goodyer
3 Woodside Avenue
London SE25 5DW

Miscellaneous

Directory of Maternity and Postnatal Care Organisations compiled by Ipswich AIMS
(from Amanda Wade, 76 Suffolk Road, Ipswich, Suffolk 1P4 2EZ (85p + 13p p&p)
Someone to Talk To Directory lists self-help and community support agencies in the
UK and the Republic of Ireland (MIND, £20).

Share Community is a charity and the only self-help clearing house, supplying details of self-help groups nationwide. They also produce Spotlight magazine which gives further details of groups. Alexandra House, 140 Battersea Park Road, London SW11 4NB (01–622 6885).

Chapter 7

Suggested reading

Why Women Don't Have Wives: Professional Success and Motherhood Terri Apter (Macmillan, 1985)

Women and Madness Phyllis Chesler (Avon Books, USA, 1973)

Living With a Toddler Brenda Crowe (Allen & Unwin, 1982)

A Woman in Your Own Right: Assertiveness and You Anne Dickson (Quartet, 1982)

The New Mother Syndrome: Coping with Postal-Natal Stress and Depression Carol Dix (Allen & Unwin, 1986, £10.95)

Help Yourself to Mental Health Mary Manning (Columbus, 1987)

The Tranquillizer Trap and How to Get Out of It Joy Melville (Fontana, 1984)

The Secret of Childhood Maria Montessori; plus other books (from The Theosophical Bookshop, 68 Great Russell Street, London WC18 3BU)

Dealing With Depression Kathy Nairne and Gerrilyn Smith (Women's Press, 1984)

Stand Your Ground: A Woman's Guide to Self-Preservation Kaleghl Quinn (Orbis/Channel 4, 1983)

Of Woman Born: Motherhood as an Experience and Institution Adrienne Rich (Virago, 1977)

Depression: The Way Out of Your Prison Dorothy Rowe (Routledge & Kegan Paul, 1983)

Depression: Its Causes and How to Overcome It Dr Caroline Shreeve (Turnstone, 1984)

The Family Bed: An Age Old Concept in Child Rearing Tine Thevenin (from ABM or LLL, see Chapter 6)

The Secret Life of the Unborn Child Dr Thomas Verny with John Kelly (Sphere, 1981)

Postnatal Depression Vivienne Welburn (Fontana, 1980)

Helpful organisations

The Institute for Complementary Medicine
21 Portland Place
London W1N 3AF
(01–636 9543)

Redwood Assertiveness Training Courses

Anne Dickson
83 Fordwych Road
London NW2 3TL
(01–452 9261)

Martial Arts Commission

First Floor Broadway House
15–16 Deptford Broadway
London SE8 4PA
(01–691 3433)

Miscellaneous

Here's Health publish a Where to Find Help directory of complementary medicine organisations each month

Index

297

Maudesley hospital, 153
Medicines, 156
Medicines: complementary, 243; herbal, 244; homeopathy, 244
Meet-a-Mum Association (MAMA), 292
Memories of Motherhood, 21
Mental health care, 145–93, 247
Mercouri, Melina, 66
Mervyn, Dr Len, 120, 127
Meyer, Dr Victor, 164
Middlesex Hospital, 164
Midwives: role in childbirth, 56–8; treatment of PND, 169–71
Miller, 113
Mills, Maggie, 64, 191
Mind and body therapy, 165–6
MIND (National Association for Mental Health), 158, 160
Mindell, Earl, 103
Miscarriage Association, 291
Montessori, Maria, 272
Mood changing: exercise, 240–41; dealing with tension, 241; music, 241; physical relaxation, 241–2; mental relaxation, 242
Mother and Baby, 204
Mother Knot, The, 58, 277
Mothering, 269, 272–3
Motherhood, 65–76; as factor in PND, 22–3; the Stepford Wives Syndrome, 66–7; disappointments, 67–8; giving up work, 68–9; new responsibilities, 69–70; love or indifference for babies, 70–71; breastfeeding, 71;

pressure to be superwoman, 71–2, 73; social isolation, 73–4; exhaustion, 74–6; a happy progression, 274–9
Motherhood and Mental Illness, 15, 171
Mothers' attitudes, 234–79; running the home, 238; taking care, 238–9; clear the decks, 239; housework, 239; shopping, 239; feeding yourself, 239–40; mood changing, 240–43; preparing for parenthood, 244–6; working for change, 246–50; self-transformation, 250–51; positive thinking, 255–61; thinking about suicide, 261; avoiding depression, 262–5; opening your mind, 264; partners in care, 265–8; loving our children, 268–74; motherhood: a happy progression, 274–9
Mothers Talking About Postnatal Depression, 3, 210
Mullins, Pauline, 83–4
Music, 241

Nairne, Kathy, 82, 158, 160, 164, 165, 261
National Advisory Committee on Nutritional Education (NANCE), 118–19
National Association for Mental Health (MIND), 158, 160, 289
National Association of Parents of Sleepless Children, 222

Society, 217–19, 230, 290
Pain relief in childbirth, 42–4
Palmer, Dr Robert, 158
Panuthos, Claudia, 257
Paper Doctors, 145
Parenthood: being a wife, 77; finances, 77–8; heavy responsibility of, 78–9; role division, 79–80; parenting arrangements, 80–81; propping up husbands, 81–2; sexual problems, 82–4
Parenting arrangements, 80–81
Parents magazine, 37, 46, 47, 79, 223, 230
Parish, Peter, 156
Partners, 199–200; in care, 265–8
Partners in Care: Puerperal Depression, 177
Paterson, Jane, 171
Patients' Association, 54, 141
Penfield, Kedzie, 166
Pfeiffer, Dr Carl, 126, 129
Philpotts, Carol, 213
Physical health, 236–7
Physical or emotional exhaustion, 254
Picardie, Justine, 232
Pithers, David, 270
Pitts, Dr Brice, 11, 15, 19, 20, 177
Placenta, 114; delivery of, 47–9; eating of, 109–10, 129
Playfair, Dr Ronald, 13
Playforth, Sarah, 228
Popplestone, Gerry, 85
Positive thinking, 255–61
Post-natal depression (PND), xviii–xx, 5–8, 21, 142, 143, 153, 156, 157, 158, 159, 163; causes, 1–2; lack of information, 2; getting recognition, understanding and treatment, 3; personal recollections of, 4–10; various manifestations of, 4–10; professional arguments, 10–24; differences in incidence, 11–12; conflicting opinions concerning, 15–19; biochemical elements in, 20; possible origins, 20–23; stresses in, 21–2, 230–32, 280–82; motherhood, 22; childbonding problems linked with, 23–4; risk factors, 24–5; factors not associated with incidence of, 25–6; guilt feelings, 63; fatigue, 74; not all in the mind, 101–4; hormonal factors, 104–6; Dalton's theories and methods, 106–8; premenstrual syndrome, 107, 109; eating the placenta, 109–10, 129; breastfeeding, 110–12; contraceptive pill, 112–13; sensitivity to hormones, 113–14; thyroid and adrenal involvement, 114–15; treatment of, 168–76, 178; prevention of, 176–81; diagnosis of, 178–80; help for, 194–5, 195–7, 200–4, 206–7, 209–13; symptoms, 195–6, 280–81; practical assistance, 197; listening to problems, 198–9; partners, 199–200; support

Rippere, Dr Vicky, 153
Rite of passage, 60; in childbirth, 28–31, 32
Ritual practices in childbirth, 30–35
Robertson, Joann, 217, 230–31
Robinson, Jean, 54, 141
Robson, Dr Kay, 23, 169
Role division, 79–80
Rolfing, 166
Romeo, Catherine, 257
Rothera, Mrs Ellen, 136
Running the home, 238
Rowe, Albert, 134
Rowe, Dorothy, 149, 198, 202
Royal College of General Practitioners, 174, 175
Royal College of Midwives, 170
Royal College of Nursing, 175

Safety and technology in childbirth, 35–7
Sagovsky, R., 178
Samaritans, 165, 289
Sandler, Professor Merton, 16, 133
Sanjack, Marion, 187
Satisfaction in childbirth, 37–8
Schizophrenia Association of Great Britain, 140
Seaman, Barbara, 126
Seaman, Gideon, 126
Secret of Childhood, The, 272
Seel, Richard, 30, 32, 33, 87–9
Selenium, 124
Self-fulfilment, 95–6
Self-Help Centre, 205
Self-transformation, 250–51
Sensitive Midwifery, 57
Sensitivity to hormones, 113–14
Sexual problems, 82–4, 90

Sexual relations, 202
Sharing the birth, 86–7
Sharpe, Sue, 21, 64
Sheffield Post-Natal Depression Support Group, 213–15, 216
Sherrat, Stella, 232
Shopping, 239
Simmons, Sheila, 162–3
Single parenthood, 89–91
Smith, Gerrilyn, 82, 158, 160, 164, 165
Smith, Sue, 212
Social factors: isolation, 73–4; poisons, 143, 144; stress as factor in PND, 21–2
Society Against Depression (SAD), 216
Society for Reproductive and Infant Psychology, 2
Society to Support Home Confinement, 285
Sokol, Robert, 29
Special care baby units, 49–50
Special needs, 219
Squatting Birth, 45
Standing Conference on Drug Abuse, 157
Stanley, Jan, 170
Stepford Wives Syndrome, 66–7, 151, 152
Stevenson, Janet, 215–16
Stewart, Nancy, 48
Stillbirth, 184
Stillbirth and Neonatal Death Society, 292
Stillbirth and Perinatal Death Association, 227
Stilwell, Barbara, 175
Stocks, Vivienne, 204
Stress, 130, 136, 143, 144, 195,